Critical Reading Questions
the MRCGP 2e

Critical Reading Questions for the MRCGP 2e

Ese Stacey MBBS, MRCGP, DCH, DRCOG, Msc Sport Med.

General Practice Educator and Sports Physician, East Sussex

and

Yinkori Toun MBBS, MRCGP, MRCP (UK), DPH (Cantab)

General Practitioner, London

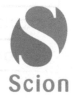

Scion

Second edition first published 2005

First edition published 1997 © BIOS Scientific Publishers Ltd
Reprinted 1999, 2001, 2002
Reprinted 2004 © Scion Publishing Ltd

ISBN 1 904842 08 9

Scion Publishing Limited
Bloxham Mill, Barford Road, Bloxham, Oxfordshire OX15 4FF
www.scionpublishing.com

Important Note from the Publisher
The information contained within this book was obtained by Scion Publishing Limited from sources believed by us to be reliable. However, while every effort has been made to ensure its accuracy, no responsibility for loss or injury whatsoever occasioned to any person acting or refraining from action as a result of information contained herein can be accepted by the authors or publishers.

The reader should remember that medicine is a constantly evolving science and while the authors and publishers have ensured that all dosages, applications and practices are based on current indications, there may be specific practices which differ between communities. You should always follow the guidelines laid down by the manufacturers of specific products and the relevant authorities in the country in which you are practising.

Production Editor: Clare Boomer
Typeset by Phoenix Photosetting, Chatham, Kent, UK
Printed by Biddles Ltd, King's Lynn, UK, www.biddles.co.uk

CONTENTS

ABBREVIATIONS

ARR	absolute risk reduction
BHS	British Hypertension Society
CSM	Committee on Safety of Medicines
'DNA'	did not attend
HRT	hormone replacement therapy
NNT	numbers needed to treat
NSAID	non-steroidal anti-inflammatory drug
OR	odds ratio
PPA	Prescription Pricing Authority
RR	relative risk
SSRI	selective serotonin re-uptake inhibitor
TCA	tricyclic antidepressant
WHO	World Health Organisation

PREFACE

During my revision for the MRCGP examination, I realized that there was a dearth of useful books to see me through the critical reading section of the exam. I decided that I would attempt to fill this gap by co-writing a book specifically aimed at MRCGP candidates as well as GP trainers. My co-author, Yinkori Toun, has been essential in giving the book some depth, particularly in the areas of critical appraisal and public health. In this latest edition, we have completely revised the material on bias and guidelines, in addition to updating many other parts of the book.

The aim of this new edition of the book continues to be to take the uninitiated candidate by the hand and lead her/him on an exploratory tour of all the major areas covered by the exam. This tour is encompassed in Part I of the book. We have used a question and answer format to expose any glaring holes in the candidate's knowledge and also to give the candidate a feel for the time constraints and pressures of actually sitting the exam. The answers are given at the end of each section.

The questions have been tested on around 30 GP registrars, who were themselves studying for the exam. Some of the answers are given as 'consensus' answers and are a collation of those from this group of registrars.

Part II of the book looks at the conceptually more difficult areas of 'Risk' and 'Numbers needed to treat (NNT)'. This section may be useful for trainers as well as GP registrars. Knowledge of these areas is essential in order to gain a complete understanding of research and critical appraisal. Screening often crops up in the exam and NNT is emerging as an important tool in general practice for communicating 'risk' to the patient.

Part III is a quick-glance revision section. Its aim is to remind the candidate of the essentials on the eve of the exam.

Ese Stacey
Yinkori Toun

PART I

- Pre-exam teaser
- Study design
- Critical appraisal
- Data interpretation
- Guidelines

PRE-EXAM TEASER

- The pre-exam teaser is designed to give you a taste of things to come.
- Give yourself 15 minutes (in total) for Sections I, II and III.
- Read all the questions before you begin your answers.

Section I

(a) Proportion of true positives that are correctly identified by the test
(b) Proportion of patients with positive test results who are correctly diagnosed
(c) Proportion of true negatives that are correctly identified by the test
(d) Proportion of patients with a positive test who are incorrectly diagnosed
(e) Proportion of patients with a negative test who are incorrectly diagnosed
(f) Proportion of patients with negative tests who are correctly diagnosed

QUESTIONS

1. From (a) to (f) above choose the statement which best fits with the words given below:
   (i) positive predictive value
   (ii) negative predictive value
   (iii) specificity
   (iv) sensitivity

Your answer ....

2. Write out a summary of the British Hypertension Society guidelines for hypertension.

Your answer ....

Section II

QUESTIONS

1. List the points to be discussed when analysing the following sections of a quantitative scientific paper:
   (a) Introduction
   (b) Methods
   (c) Results
   (d) Discussion

Your answer ....

2. List the points to be discussed when analysing guidelines.

Your answer ....

3. Give a short description of the following types of study:
   (a) Case-control
   (b) Cross-sectional
   (c) Randomised
   (d) Controlled

Your answer ....

Section III

1. Do not answer question 2 of Section I.

Answers

Section I

Answer to question 1

(i) b
(ii) f
(iii) c
(iv) a

- *Sensitivity* is the proportion of true positives that are correctly identified by the test.
- *Specificity* is the proportion of true negatives that are correctly identified by the test.
- *Positive predictive value* is the proportion of patients with positive test results who are correctly diagnosed.
- *Negative predictive value* is the proportion of patients with negative tests who are correctly diagnosed.

The predictive values of a test depend on the prevalence of the abnormality in the population of patients being tested. The prevalence in clinical practice may differ from the prevalence in a published study. If the prevalence of the disease is low the positive predictive value will be low even if both sensitivity and specificity are high.

Answer to question 2

Section III says 'Do not answer' this question! **Read all the questions before attempting your answers.**

Section II

Answer to question 1

Introduction

- Background
- Aims
- Relevance
- Originality

Background: The background to the study is given first.

Aims: The aims of the study should then be clearly stated.

Relevance: The study should be relevant to (in our case) general practice.

Originality: The idea behind the study should be original.

Methods

- Design
- Outcome measures
- Subjects

Design: The design of the study should be appropriate for its aims. The study should be repeatable. All the instruments (including questionnaires) should be validated and reliable. Confounding variables should be considered and dealt with accordingly.

Outcome measures: Appropriate outcome measures should be selected which are consistent with the aims and design of the study.

Subjects: Subjects should be representative of the population in question. Controls may or may not have been used in the study. Is the use of controls appropriate? The selection of subjects and controls should be appropriate and without bias. The numbers involved in the study should be enough to detect a statistically significant result.

Results

- Understandable
- Response rate
- Drop-outs
- Statistical analysis

Understandable: The results, including tables and graphs, should be clear and easy to understand.

Response rate: The response rate should be mentioned where appropriate (e.g. the number of questionnaires completed).

Drop-outs: If possible, the characteristics of drop-outs, non-attenders and those who fail to respond should be defined.

Statistics: The statistical analysis used should be clear and appropriate for the design of the study.

Discussion

- Critical evaluation of results
- Conclusion
- Applicability

Critical evaluation of results: The results should be discussed critically. The author should point out possible areas of bias, error or limitation. Results should be discussed with respect to other literature.

Conclusion: The author's conclusion should be consistent with the results of the study.

Applicability: Are the results applicable to your population? Are the results of the study likely to change your clinical practice?

Others

- Title, author, institute, journal
- Writing style
- Ethics
- References
- Conflicts of interest

Title, author, institute and journal: These may give the reader some idea of how relevant and robust the study is.

Writing style: The paper should be easy to read and understand.

Ethics: Some studies have ethical considerations. These should have been taken into account and approval from the local ethics committee should be sought.

References: These should be appropriate and up-to-date.

Conflicts of interest: Some journals now acknowledge any possible conflict of interest, one of which can be the source of funding for the study.

Answer to question 2

See Part I, Guidelines, pp. 77–83

Answer to question 3

See Part I, Study design, pp. 13–34.

Comment

I hope that this pre-exam teaser has got you in the mood for some exam study. It may have highlighted some of your deficiencies, especially the 'do not answer' question and the question concerning sensitivity, specificity, and predictive values. Don't worry! We'll take you through it all, bit by bit, and by the end of the book the cold sweats and palpitations will have ceased! Happy reading!

STUDY DESIGN

- The randomised controlled trial is seen as the gold standard in terms of strength of evidence. This type of study is, of course, not always practical and may be unethical in certain situations. Although other types of study are less robust, understanding their strengths and weaknesses will help you to form appropriate conclusions from the results.

- This section contains questions that provide an introduction to study design.

- For questions 1–4 you are presented with part of a published article. Read the article before answering the question. Questions 5–10 are further extended matching questions with in-depth answers, which will give you a little more information about study design.

- The main categories of study methods are covered here. This is followed by a statistical section.

EXTENDED MATCHING QUESTIONS

- Read papers 1–4. After reading each paper, answer the corresponding question on p. 21.

Paper 1: ... study of endogenous sex hormones and fatal cardiovascular disease in postmenopausal women

Elizabeth Barrett-Connor and Deborah Goodman-Gruen
British Medical Journal (1995) **311**: 1193–1196.
Reproduced with permission from the BMJ Publishing Group.

METHODS

Between 1972 and 1974 all adult residents in Rancho Bernardo, California, were invited to participate in a study of risk factors for cardiovascular disease, and 82% did so. Participants were seen between 7 30 and 11 00 am after a requested 12 hour fast. A standardised questionnaire was completed which included questions about personal and family history of heart disease (heart attack or heart failure), history of cigarette smoking, and current use of oestrogen. Blood pressure was measured with a mercury sphygmomanometer after the participant had been seated for at least five minutes. Height and weight were measured with the participants wearing lightweight clothing without shoes; body mass index (weight (kg)/height (m)^2) was used to estimate obesity. Total plasma cholesterol concentration was measured in a Centers for Disease Control standardised lipid research clinic laboratory with an AutoAnalyzer; lipoprotein concentrations were not determined at baseline. Fasting plasma glucose concentration was measured in a hospital diagnostic laboratory with a hexokinase method. Plasma for endogenous sex hormone assays was obtained and frozen at $-70\,°C$.

Between 1984 and 1986 sex hormones were measured in an endocrinology research laboratory (S S C Yen) by radioimmunoassay with thawed specimens obtained from postmenopausal women at the 1972–4 venepuncture[9]. Previous work in this laboratory demonstrated no hormone deterioration over 15 years when samples were frozen and stored in tightly sealed containers. Bioavailable testosterone and bioavailable oestradiol were determined by using a method modified from Tremblay and Dube.[10] The sensitivity and the between and within assay coefficients of variation, respectively, were 1.8 nmol/1 (30 pg/ml), 4% and 8% for androstenedione;

0.1 nmol/1 (25 pg/ml), 4% and 10% for testosterone; 26 pmol/1 (7 pg/ml), 15% and 16% for oestrone; 18 pmol/1 (5 pg/ml), 8% and 12% for oestradiol; 0.03 nmol/1 (8 pg/ml), 5.8% and 6.0% for bioavailable testosterone and 4 pmol/1 (1 pg/ml), 3.7% and 4.2% for bioavailable oestradiol. Six women with oestradiol concentrations and three with oestrone concentrations below the sensitivity of the assay were excluded from these analyses, as were women who reported use of oestrogen at baseline (n=302). All oestradiol and oestrone concentrations were consistent with post-menopausal status.

Vital status was determined annually for 99.9% of the cohort to 1992, a 19 year follow up. Death certificates, obtained for all those who died, were coded for underlying cause of death by a certified nosologist using the *International Classification of Diseases*, adapted ninth revision (ICD-9). Cardiovascular disease included codes 400 to 438 and ischaemic heart disease codes 410 to 414. Review of medical records by a panel of cardiologists in a 30% sample of those whose death certificates included a diagnosis of fatal cardiovascular disease confirmed the diagnosis in 85%.

Data were analysed by using SAS.[11] Logarithms of hormone concentrations were used for analysis to account for slightly skewed distributions. Results were similar for untransformed data, which are shown here. Age adjusted mean hormone concentrations were compared between women with and without known heart disease at baseline. All other analyses excluded women with prevalent heart disease. Pearson's partial correlation coefficients were calculated to assess the strength of the association between the hormones and risk factors for cardiovascular disease. Mean hormone concentrations adjusted for age were compared for high and low risk categories of coronary heart disease by using analysis of covariance. The independent contribution of the measured hormones, age, systolic blood pressure, diastolic blood pressure, plasma cholesterol concentration, fasting plasma glucose, obesity, and cigarette smoking to the risk of death from cardiovascular disease or ischaemic heart disease was assessed by using Cox's proportional hazards model.[12] All P values are two tailed. No adjustment was made for multiple comparisons; instead, exact P values are shown in the tables: in the text the term significance refers to $P < 0.05$ or 95% confidence intervals that do not include one.

[9] Anderson DC, Hopper BR, Lasley BL, Yen SSC. A simple method for the assay of eight steroids in small volumes of plasma. *Steroids* 1976; 28: 179–96.
[10] Tremblay RR, Dube JY. Plasma concentrations of free and non-TeBG bound testosterone in women on oral contraceptives. *Contraception* 1974; 10: 599–605.
[11] SAS Institute. SAS user's guide. Version 6.03. Cary: North Carolina: SAS Institute, 1985.
[12] Cox DR. Regression models and life-tables. *Journal of the Royal Statistical Society (B)* 1972; 34: 187–220.

Paper 2: Utilisation of hormone replacement therapy by women doctors

A.J. Isaacs, A.R. Britton and Klim McPherson

British Medical Journal (1995) **311**: 1399–1401.

METHODS

Sampling—The sampling frame consisted of all women doctors who obtained full registration with the General Medical Council between 1952 and 1976 inclusive and whose names appeared on the principal list of the *Medical Register* in 1993. A randomised sample of 1550 was taken, stratified by five year bands, to obtain an approximately even age distribution across the age range 40 to 65 years. Of these, 36 living abroad were excluded, giving a final sample size of 1514.

Questionnaire—A postal questionnaire, explanatory letter, and reply paid envelope were sent to all doctors in the sample in June 1993. Initial non-responders were sent a reminder letter, and finally a further letter with a second copy of the questionnaire and another reply paid envelope was sent in July. All responses received by the end of 1993 were coded and the data entered onto a computerised database. Statistical analyses were carried out with Epi-Info.[5] When answers to specific questions were missing these respondents were omitted from the relevant analyses. The questionnaire covered various demographic and behavioural factors which will be reported fully elsewhere, the current report being restricted to the prevalence and duration of use of hormone replacement therapy.

[5]Dean AG, Dean JA, Burton AH, Dicker RC. Epi Info. Version 5. Stone Mountain, GA, USA: 1990.

(see following page for Table II from this paper)

TABLE II—Prevalence of use of hormone replacement therapy by age group in women doctors*

	Current use		Ever use		Total
	No of women	% (95% Confidence interval)	No of women	% (95% Confidence interval)	
All women					
All ages	344	28.4 (25.9 to 30.9)	480	39.6 (36.8 to 42.4)	1211
Age group (years):					
40–44	9	6.4 (2.3 to 10.5)	11	7.9 (3.4 to 12.4)	140
45–49	49	21.2 (15.9 to 26.5)	55	23.8 (18.3 to 29.3)	231
50–54	85	43.3 (36.5 to 50.2)	109	55.6 (48.6 to 62.6)	196
55–59	114	44.9 (38.8 to 51.0)	155	61.0 (55.0 to 67.0)	254
60–64	71	26.0 (20.8 to 31.2)	117	42.9 (37.0 to 48.8)	273
65–69	14	15.4 (8.0 to 22.8)	28	30.8 (21.3 to 40.3)	91
70–	2	7.7 (0.0 to 17.9)	5	19.2 (4.1 to 34.3)	26
Excluding premenopausal women					
All ages	344	37.8 (34.6 to 41.0)	472	51.9 (48.7 to 55.1)	909
Age groups (years)					
40–44	9	52.9 (29.2 to 76.6)	11	64.7 (42.0 to 87.4)	17
45–49	49	54.4 (43.2 to 64.7)	52	57.8 (47.6 to 68.0)	90
50–54	85	53.5 (45.7 to 61.3)	104	65.4 (58.0 to 72.8)	159
55–59	114	45.1 (39.0 to 51.2)	155	61.3 (55.3 to 67.3)	253
60–64	71	26.0 (20.8 to 31.2)	117	42.9 (37.0 to 48.8)	273
65–69	14	15.4 (8.0 to 22.8)	28	30.8 (21.3 to 40.3)	91
70–	22	7.7 (0.0 to 17.9)	5	19.2 (4.1 to 34.3)	26

* Fourteen respondents who did not state their date of birth were allocated to the most probable group according to year of registration.

Paper 3: Cigarette smoking, tar yields, and non-fatal myocardial infarction: . . . in the United Kingdom
S. Parish, R. Collins, R. Peto, L. Youngman, J. Barton, K. Jayne, R. Clarke, P. Appleby, V. Lyon, S. Cederholm-Williams, J. Marshall, P. Sleight for the International Studies of Infarct Survival (ISIS) Collaborators
British Medical Journal (1995) **311**: 471–477
Reproduced with permission from the BMJ Publishing Group.

METHODS AND RESULTS

Cases were the survivors in the United Kingdom aged 30–79 from the ISIS-3 or ISIS-4 trials who completed an epidemiological questionnaire sent to them a few months after their infarction. Those who were asked to complete it were all the survivors from ISIS-3, but ISIS-4 only the survivors aged 30–59 who on admission to hospital were reported to be cigarette smokers. Thus, although only cases from ISIS-3 can be used to compare smokers with non-smokers, the cases from ISIS-4 strengthen the analyses of tar yields among smokers aged 30–59. The ISIS-3 questionnaire asked the cases to identify all their brothers, sisters, and children aged at least 30 who were resident in the United Kingdom. A similar 'control' questionnaire was then sent to such relatives, accompanied by a second copy, which the relatives, if married, were to ask their spouse to complete. One reminder was sent to cases and relatives who did not reply, and inconsistencies or omissions were queried once.

Of the 20681 ISIS-3 patients in the United Kingdom, 19065 who were not known to be dead were posted the case questionnaire, of whom 1346 were found to be dead and 13969 (79% of presumed survivors) completed it. The control questionnaire was sent to 30247 relatives of ISIS-3 cases, of whom 75 were found to be dead and 21995 (73% of presumed survivors) and 14245 of their spouses completed it. Patients with a history of stroke, gastrointestinal bleeding, or ulcer tended not to have been recruited into the ISIS-3 trial,[19] and so people with such conditions were not eligible as cases or controls. Of those who completed questionnaires, 2002 cases and 3851 controls were excluded because they were under 30, over 79, or of unknown age or because they had a self reported history of 'definite stroke' or of 'bleeding or ulcer in (or near) the stomach.'

ISIS-4 patients in the United Kingdom aged 30–59 who were described at trial entry as current smokers were also sent the questionnaire. The response rate for such patients was similar in both trials. Any of these ISIS-4 patients whose questionnaire response indicated that they were not cigarette smokers at the time of their infarction were excluded. ISIS-4 (and, to some extent, ISIS-3) tended to exclude patients with shock or persistent hypotension,[20] but such exclusions should not bias the epidemiological analyses of tobacco use.

[19] ISIS-3 (Third International Study of Infarct Survival) Collaborative Group. ISIS-3: A randomised trial of streptokinase vs tissue plasminogen activator vs anistreplase and of aspirin plus heparin vs aspirin alone among 41,299 cases of suspected acute myocardial infarction. *Lancet* 1992; 339: 753–70.

[20] ISIS-4 (Fourth International Study of Infarct Survival) Collaborative Group. ISIS-4: A randomised factorial trial assessing early oral captopril, oral mononitrate, and intravenous magnesium sulphate in 58,050 patients with suspected acute myocardial infarction. *Lancet* 1995; 345: 669–85.

TABLE II—*Non-fatal myocardial infarction: age-specific effect of cigarette use in people with no history of major neoplastic or vascular disease*

Age (years)	Current smoker of manufactured cigarettes only		Non-smoker with no regular cigarette use in past 10 years		Myocardial infarction*	
	Cases	Controls	Cases	Controls	Risk ratio (95% confidence interval)	Test statistic†
30–39	78	1784	35	4873	6.33 (4.22 to 9.51)	8.9
40–49	293	1497	190	4306	4.66 (3.82 to 5.69)	15.1
50–59	435	861	508	2701	3.10 (2.64 to 3.65)	13.7
30–59	806	4142	733	11880	3.85 (3.41 to 4.34)	22.1
60–69	416	653	707	2299	2.54 (2.16 to 2.98)	11.3
70–79	111	163	369	942	1.92 (1.45 to 2.54)	4.6
60–79	527	816	1076	3241	2.37 (2.06 to 2.72)	12.1

* Smoker v non-smoker rates standardised for age and sex.
† Number of standard deviations by which the logarithm of the risk ratio differs from zero.

Paper 4: Cardiac and vascular morbidity in women receiving adjuvant tamoxifen for breast cancer in a randomised trial

Carolyn C. McDonald, Freda E. Alexander, Bruce W. Whyte, A. Patrick Forrest, Helen J. Steward, for the Scottish Cancer Trials Breast Group
British Medical Journal (1995) **311**: 977–980.
Reproduced with permission from the BMJ Publishing Group.

PATIENTS AND METHODS

Between 1978 and 1984, 1312 eligible women with primary operable breast cancer were entered into the Scottish adjuvant tamoxifen trial. Of these, 242 (18%) were premenopausal, being within one year of their last menstrual period. Women in the treatment arm of the trial received tamoxifen 20 mg daily for five years after their mastectomy (or until earlier relapse); women in the control arm did not receive adjuvant tamoxifen, but this was to be given for treatment of later relapse of disease. Women in the treatment arm who were alive and still free of relapse at five years were offered further randomisation either to stop tamoxifen treatment or to continue taking it until relapse or death. Information on recurrence and death was sought annually.

No baseline data were available for factors not considered relevant to survival from breast cancer. In particular information on smoking, blood lipids, weight, and blood pressure (important factors in cardiovascular morbidity) was not collected.

In designing the present study, we decided to include all eligible women rather than just postmenopausal women as previously[1] because our intention was to examine a range of potential health related effects and the inclusion of younger women would not increase the incidence of myocardial infarction itself.

DATA LINKAGE

A computerised linkage program at Information and Statistics Division attempted to identify episodes in the computerised inpatient record scheme for all trial patients for the period from 1 January 1978 to 31 December 1992. Surname, forename, date of birth, date of mastectomy, and date of death (if appropriate) were used as matching items. A probability based score was used to measure the likelihood of two records matching. The odds of a correct match were calculated for each variable and multiplied together to give the overall probability that the two records belonged to the same person. The threshold value was kept low to minimise the risk of true matches being rejected.

In the Scottish cancer trials office each matching pair of records was checked. For each confirmed match, the date of admission and code of cause[3] (other than those related to breast cancer) were added to the existing trial database. This included dates of patients' birth, randomisation, local and systemic relapse, and death. Allocated treatment and its duration were entered for all trial subjects. From the resulting database all the above items except locoregional relapse alone were extracted for the analysis. Table I shows the causes of hospital admissions considered in this report. These categories were defined before the data were inspected. Because of the small numbers involved, deep vein thrombosis and pulmonary embolus were analysed as a single group of thromboembolic events. Most of the subjects admitted to hospital for both deep vein thrombosis and pulmonary embolism had identical dates for the two; when they differed the earlier of the two dates was taken as the date of the thromboembolic event.

(see following page for Table I from this paper)

TABLE 1—*Causes of hospital admissions included in study and numbers of cases analysed and of cases rejected because of presence of systemic cancer*

International Classification of Diseases, Ninth Revision[3]		No of cases	
Description	Code	Analysed	Excluded
Myocardial infarction	410	37	9
Cerebrovascular disease	430–437	45	7
Pulmonary embolism or phlebitis and thrombophlebitis	4151, 451	25	10
Other ischaemic heart diseases	411–414	42	10

[1] McDonald CC, Stewart HJ, for the Scottish Breast Cancer Committee. Fatal myocardial infarction in the Scottish adjuvant tamoxifen trial. *BMJ* 1991; 303: 435–7.

[3] International classification of diseases, ninth revision Geneva: World Health Organisation, 1978.

EXTENDED MATCHING QUESTIONS

(a)   Retrospective
(b)   Prospective
(c)   Case-control
(d)   Cross-sectional survey
(e)   Randomised controlled

For each question below, choose a letter from (a) to (e) which best describes the paper given. Only one answer for each question is correct. Read the question and paper carefully before answering.

QUESTIONS

1.   Paper 1: How would you describe this study?
2.   Paper 2: What kind of study is this?
3.   Paper 3: This is a retrospective study; how else might you describe it?
4.   Paper 4: How might you best describe this study?

Your answers ....

EXTENDED MATCHING QUESTIONS

Answers

Answer to question 1

The study starts in the early 1970s and ends 19 years later, which means that it must be a prospective study. A series of observations were made on the subjects. There is nothing to suggest that it is randomised or controlled. Therefore, the answer is (b).

Answer to question 2

The title of the paper gives some indication of the design of the study. The table of results gives the prevalence of use of hormone replacement therapy (HRT), which is another clue to the answer. A random sample of women doctors who were registered with the General Medical Council between 1952 and 1976 were asked if they used HRT. This was a cross-sectional study. The answer is (d).

Answer to question 3

This is a case-control study. Cases are patients who have sustained and survived an acute myocardial infarction (MI). Controls are their nominated relatives aged 30 and above. Similar exclusion criteria are applied in selecting cases and controls. A questionnaire is used to measure smoking histories, the exposure of interest. The risk of an MI in current smokers is compared to that in non-smokers for different agebands, to give risk ratios (relative risks). The answer is (c).

Answer to question 4

This is a clinical trial. Clinical trials tend to be randomised or controlled or both. It is not very clear but women seem to be randomised either to receive tamoxifen treatment or to receive no adjuvant treatment (in which case they are controls). Those women who have been taking tamoxifen (and are still alive after 5 years) are further randomised to either stop or continue taking tamoxifen. This is a randomised control trial. Some may have been tempted to simply state that this is a prospective study but the question asks 'How might you *best* describe the study?' The answer is (e).

MORE QUESTIONS ON STUDY DESIGN

EXTENDED MATCHING QUESTIONS

(a) Retrospective
(b) Prospective
(c) Case-control
(d) Cohort
(e) Cross-sectional survey
(f) Randomised controlled
(g) Randomised

QUESTIONS

What type of study do the following statements describe? Choose from (a) to (g) shown above. There is only one correct answer for each question.

5. Prevalence of condition can be assessed but the incidence cannot. The exact timing of the exposure cannot be assessed.
6. An intervention study which, if designed well, can give good evidence of cause and effect. Subjects receiving a treatment can be compared with those not receiving a treatment.
7. Its optimal use is for uncommon exposures and several outcomes can be studied. The incidence of the disease can be assessed and selection bias is less likely.
8. A descriptive study which provides a 'snapshot' of the population in question.
9. Its optimal use is for uncommon diseases. Multiple exposures for a single disease can be studied. Few subjects are required and the studies are usually quick and easy.
10. Put the following methods of design in order of increasing strength of evidence of causality:

experimental, case-control, cohort

Your answers ....

MORE QUESTIONS ON STUDY DESIGN

Answers

Answer to question 5

(e)

Answer to question 6

(f)

Answer to question 7

(d)

Answer to question 8

(e)

Answer to question 9

(c)

Answer to question 10

(1) Case-control
(2) Cohort
(3) Experimental

TYPES OF STUDY DESIGN

CROSS-SECTIONAL SURVEYS

These descriptive studies are sometimes called **prevalence** studies. They look at data from a particular point in time and therefore represent a 'snapshot' of the population in question. The presence or absence of disease can be assessed to give the prevalence. These findings can be compared with other data collected at the same time, such as age, sex or body weight. These comparisons may suggest a hypothesis which can be tested using other types of study.

CASE-CONTROL STUDIES

- Subjects already have the disease in question and are called 'cases'. Controls are taken from the same population as the cases but do not have the disease.

- The past history of the subjects is examined to look for 'exposure' to an agent or the presence of a factor which may cause or be associated with the disease. 'Exposure' is usually assessed by questionnaire, interview or looking through medical records.

- Case-control studies are used to investigate a hypothesis and may be followed up by cohort or intervention studies.

- They are also known as **retrospective** (i.e. they look back).

- The incidence of the disease in the population cannot be calculated.

- The true relative risk and the attributable risk cannot be calculated. An estimate of the relative risk can be calculated. This is called the odds ratio.

- The relative risk can only be estimated from the odds ratio **if:**

  (a) the incidence of the disease in the general population is low (less than 5%).
  (b) the control group is representative of the general population.
  (c) cases and controls are free from selection bias. An example of this bias occurs when we look at the risk of cardiovascular disease in women using HRT. The kind of women who undergo this therapy tend to be self-selected (affluent, health-conscious) so that the risk of them developing cardiovascular disease will be lower than in the general population.

Advantages of case-control studies

- Small numbers of subjects can be used.
- They are useful for looking at rare conditions.
- Compared to cohort studies they can be performed quickly with minimal expense.
- Multiple exposures can be studied.

Disadvantages of case-control studies

- They are retrospective.
  - (a) Recall of past events can cause difficulties. Subjects with the disease are often better at recalling past events than subjects without the disease, who may have no interest in the study (Recall-bias).
  - (b) A causal relationship may be difficult to establish with a retrospective study.
- The selection of cases and controls becomes more important with rare conditions. Overdiagnosis or underdiagnosis of the condition will make a significant impact on the results.
- The selection of controls may prove difficult.
  - (a) It may be difficult to ensure that controls come from the same population as cases.
  - (b) It may be difficult to eliminate all confounding variables.

COHORT STUDIES

These are usually **prospective** studies (i.e. they look ahead). However, beware, cohort studies can also be retrospective (not covered here). Subjects who have been exposed to a particular agent are followed up. The characteristics of those who develop the disease can then be identified. Incidence, relative risk and attributable risk can be calculated.

Advantages of cohort studies

- The results obtained from cohort studies are more robust than case-control studies.
- Methods can be standardized to reduce observer, subject and technical error.
- They are good for examining the effects of a rare exposure.
- Several outcomes can be evaluated from exposure to the same agent.
- The incidence of the disease can be calculated directly from cohort studies.

Disadvantages of cohort studies

- Causal relationships can be difficult to interpret.
- Large populations are studied over a long period of time, which means that cohort studies are expensive.
- Follow up of large populations can be difficult.

RANDOMISED CONTROLLED TRIALS

These are intervention studies. They are often prompted by the findings of observational studies (i.e. case-control, cohort or cross-sectional surveys). They are **experimental** in design. Randomisation means that they are less susceptible to confounding variables. There is usually an intervention group and a control group (although sometimes there are more than two groups). In a randomised controlled trial, subjects are allocated to one of the two groups in a random fashion. Random allocation can be performed in several ways but will not be discussed here. Randomised controlled trials, if well-designed, can give the best evidence of cause and effect.

STATISTICAL SECTION

When conducting a study, the aim is to draw conclusions about the characteristics of a general population from your sample study population. Any difference that does occur may well be due to one of four factors:

(a) Chance sampling variation
(b) Biases in the study
(c) Confounding factors
(d) True difference

The effect of the first three factors must be assessed before concluding that any difference is a true one.

BIAS

This is defined as a systematic error in the design or execution of a study that leads to an erroneous result. You can think of this as being like a design fault in a measuring instrument. There are many types of bias and certain types of study design are prone to particular types.

Selection bias is one such type that arises when a population subgroup has an unequal chance of being chosen (such as selection of cases from only single-handed practices).

Recall bias may occur when relatives or individuals with a diagnosis under investigation such as autism have a clearer memory of events leading up to the illness than their controls, a problem in case control studies.

Loss of individuals to follow up over time can lead to biases in assessing the magnitude of the final outcome. Those who have dropped out may be from a healthier more mobile population or conversely may have died of coexisting morbidity.

Observation bias can occur in those measuring end results such as a change in blood pressure or reduction in pain scores. It is desirable therefore to blind both subjects and observers to knowledge about treatment or control in intervention trials.

Unlike chance and confounding factors it is difficult to assess the effects of bias on the final outcome of a study. Well-designed research attempts to minimise its effect at the outset. The randomised double-blind controlled trial is the ideal design for reducing the effects of bias but it is by no means a guarantee of freedom from bias.

HYPOTHESIS TESTS AND *P* VALUES

When conducting a study, we are often comparing data from two groups. Any difference that is found in the data between the two groups may be due to chance variability. We can check whether the populations are truly different by performing a hypothesis (significance) test.

1. The first step involves a statement of the null hypothesis.

> The null hypothesis states that there is no difference between the two groups under study.

In other words, the two sample groups under study are from the same overall population; that is, the intervention will have no effect.

2. The next stage involves conducting a test of statistical significance based on the null hypothesis. There are various tests used depending on the type of data involved, such as the *t*-test and chi-squared test. For more details concerning these tests, you should refer to a statistics text book (e.g. Kirkwood, B.R. (1988) *Essentials of Medical Statistics*, Blackwell Scientific Publications, Oxford).

3. The value obtained from the statistical calculation leads to a *P* value.

> The *P* value is simply the probability of this result occurring by chance, if the null hypothesis were true.

If the probability is small, then the results from your study are unlikely to occur due to chance. It is thus deemed to be a statistically significant result.

4. A *P* value of less than 0.05 is usually taken to indicate statistical significance in most clinical research.

Problems with *P* values

- If the study is poorly designed, contains biases or is affected by confounding factors, the *P* values will be irrelevant. It is therefore most important to critically appraise the study, before paying attention to the *P* values.

- The *P* value is also a function of the sample size. This means that studies which are too small may not have the capacity to detect a statistically significant difference even when there is one. This is referred to as the *power* of a study. The sample size required to give sufficient *power* should be calculated at the stage of study design.

CONFIDENCE INTERVALS

Confidence intervals give you more information than *P* values. Not only can they tell you whether results are statistically significant but they can also tell you the degree of certainty about the size of a difference between two groups.

- A confidence interval is simply an estimate of any value. It tells you with a specified probability (certainty) that the true value lies within the confidence limits. The 95% confidence intervals tell you that there is a 95% chance that the true value lies within the stated limits (or 5% chance of lying outside these limits).

Example

A study quotes the change in mean cholesterol in mmol/1 between treatment and control groups. The data are presented with 95% confidence limits in brackets as:

Mean change in cholesterol = 1.5 (0.1–2.3)

This means that we can be 95% certain that the mean value lies between 0.1 and 2.3 mmol/1. Whilst a change of 2.3 mmol/1 is of relevance in clinical practice, a change of 0.1 mmol/1 is not.

If the confidence interval is very wide, this indicates considerable uncertainty around the value (greater chance variability in the sample). Narrow confidence intervals give you greater certainty (less chance variability in the sample).

- Confidence intervals can be calculated from the results of many types of study. You can calculate confidence limits for relative risks and odds ratios. The interpretation is explained in the following example.

Example

The results of cohort studies enable the calculation of relative risks (i.e. the ratio of disease incidence in the exposed groups to the incidence in non-exposed groups). A relative risk of one (RR = 1) means there is no association between the exposure and the outcome. If a study found a two-fold increase in the relative risk for bowel cancer with a high fat intake, this may be an important finding in clinical terms. The result is presented with the 95% confidence interval:

RR for bowel cancer = 2 (0.8–2.7)

This confidence interval tells you that the risk associated with high fat intake could be anything from 0.8 to 2.7 times greater than for those unexposed to a high fat intake. It is important to note that the relative risk could actually be less than 1 from this study. The fact that the range of values includes a relative risk of 1 implies that the exposure might have no effect at all. The results of this study are therefore not statistically significant.

CONFOUNDING FACTORS

In any study, the effects of chance can be assessed by performing a hypothesis test. The effects of bias can be reduced by good study design. The effect of confounding must also be considered.

> Confounding is the spurious association between two factors under study, due to a third factor.

There are many common confounding factors such as age, sex, smoking habit, race and socioeconomic group.

Example

We know from case control studies that HRT use is associated with a reduced risk of heart disease. However, the kind of women that use HRT tend to be from a high socioeconomic group. Since more affluent people also tend to be fitter this can lead to a spurious association if not taken into account.

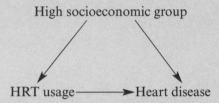

Independently of the outcome (heart disease), high socioeconomic group is also associated with greater uptake and use of HRT, the exposure under study.

In this example, socioeconomic group acts as the confounding factor. It may magnify any benefits of HRT on the occurrence of heart disease.

- Making the association more extreme is known as *positive confounding*.

- Neutralizing the degree of association is known as *negative confounding*.

There are several methods of controlling for known confounding factors. It can be done at the study design stage or during analysis of the data. These areas will not be dealt with in this book.

SYSTEMATIC REVIEWS AND META-ANALYSIS

Sometimes the results of one or more small studies lack individual power to detect a statistically significant result. It is possible to conduct a detailed, **systematic overview/review** of all the studies in a particular research area. Those studies which meet explicit quality standards and are broadly similar in design are then combined to give an overall final result. The literature search should include unpublished trials (studies with a statistically significant result are more likely to be published, leading to publication bias), as well as searching non-English databases, and contacting experts in the field.

The statistical pooling of the studies to give an overall result is known as meta-analysis. The final result can be expressed as a pooled odds ratio (OR) relative risk (RR) or Number needed to treat (NNT).

The following diagram is known as a **Forest plot** or **Blobbogram**. It displays the results of a systematic review. Four trials have been identified following a comprehensive search. They have been plotted with their individual odds ratios (blobs) and confidence intervals (horizontal lines running through the blobs) along a vertical **line of no effect** (i.e. where the OR is 0 or RR is 1). The overall pooled OR is a mathematical combination of all the studies' results and is represented by the diamond. The width of this diamond represents its confidence intervals.

Forest Plot of four trials

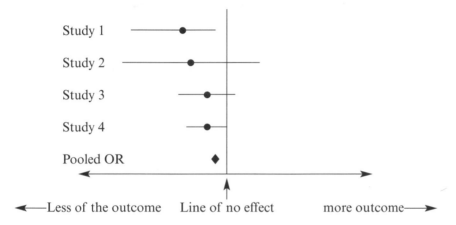

When combining studies it is important that the individual studies are broadly similar in terms of population, methodology and design. This is because what you are in effect doing is trying to approximate to a large well-designed multi-centre mega-trial which has enough statistical power to detect a significant difference, i.e. you combine smaller trials to make a bigger one.

You can assess how similar these individual small trials are in several ways. One method is to review the clinical and methodological data on included studies. Some studies may have been conducted in sicker patients in a hospital setting, so the results may not be appropriate to combine with studies conducted on community based populations.

Another method is to look at the Forest plot to see if the study results are broadly in agreement. They should lie on the same side of the 'line of no effect'. There should also be a significant overlap in their confidence intervals. If you see studies scattered across both sides of the line of no significance with no meeting of their confidence intervals then you have to question whether the researchers have in fact tried to combine apples with pears.

A more formal method of analysing how similar the trials are, is to conduct a statistical test of heterogeneity. This is often displayed as a chi-squared (x^2) test of heterogeneity with its P value. For example in a meta-analysis of ten trials a chi-squared test value of 9 with P value of 0.32 implies there is no significant heterogeneity.

In general a low P value or a chi-squared value higher than its degrees of freedom (the degrees of freedom is the number of trials included minus one) suggests significant heterogeneity. However, the chi-squared test is less than perfect, and a non-significant result does not completely exclude heterogeneity.

Finally, any sources of heterogeneity, be they clinical or methodological, should be discussed in more detail by the study authors of the systematic review.

If the Forest plot above was displaying the effect of a new drug on cardiovascular mortality we would be interested in the pooled result represented by the diamond lying to the left of the midline; this equates to less mortality with the intervention.

Archie Cochrane was a renowned epidemiologist and pioneer of the Evidence Based Medicine movement. His work led to the establishment of the first Cochrane Centre in 1992 and then the International Cochrane Collaboration in 1993. This collaboration aims to identify and disseminate the results of high quality systematic reviews regarding important areas of clinical care. Their logo represents a Forest Plot of seven trials indicating the benefits of antenatal steroids on survival in preterm labour. The accompanying explanation of the seminal work behind this logo makes an interesting read (www.cochrane.org/logo/).

CRITICAL APPRAISAL

The following questions are in exam style.

- You have 15 minutes for each question.

- Write clearly and concisely. Structure your answer. This will help you to keep focused on the question. You may wish to work through these questions with a group of fellow candidates and let someone else read your answer. This will make sure that your answer is legible. Remember, if the examiner can't read your writing, you won't get any marks.

- The answers are 'consensus' answers and are collated from the answers of around 30 GP registrars.

CRITICAL APPRAISAL

48 HOURS' BED REST FOR BACK PAIN

Does 48 hours' bed rest influence the outcome of acute low back pain?
M.J.B. Wilkinson
British Journal of General Practice (1995) **September:** 481.
Reproduced with permission from the *British Journal of General Practice*.

SUMMARY

Background. Bed rest is a traditional treatment for back pain, yet only in recent years has the therapeutic benefit of this been questioned.
Aim. The aim of this pilot study was to ascertain whether or not 48 hours' bed rest had an effect on the outcome of acute low back pain.
Method. The study was conducted as a randomised controlled trial to compare a prescription of 48 hours' strict bed rest with controls; the control subjects were encouraged to remain mobile and to have no daytime rest. Nine general practitioners from practices in the West Midlands recruited patients in the age range 16–60 years who presented with low back pain of less than seven days' duration, with or without pain radiation. The outcome measures assessed were: change in straight leg raise and lumbar flexion after seven days, Oswestry and Roland-Morris disability scores after seven days and 28 days, and time taken from work.
Results. Forty two patients were recruited: 20 were allocated to bed rest and 22 as controls. Compared with the bed rest group the control group had statistically better Roland-Morris scores at day seven ($P < 0.05$) but not at day 28. At day seven, there were no statistically significant differences between groups in straight leg raise or lumbar flexion measurements although the control group had a better mean lumbar flexion than the bed rest group. The improvement in disability scores at day seven compared with day one was similar for the two groups but more of the control group had fully recovered (defined as scores of one or zero on the Roland-Morris disability scale and five or less on the Oswestry disability scale) by day seven. Remaining mobile did not appear to cause any adverse effects. The number of days lost from work in both groups was equal. A large number of self-remedies and physical therapies were recorded by subjects from both groups.
Conclusion. The results of this pilot study did not indicate whether bed rest or remaining mobile was superior for the treatment of low back pain; however, the study sample was small. Subjects in the control group possibly

fared better as they appeared to have better lumbar flexion at day seven. It appears that 48 hours' bed rest cannot be recommended for the treatment of acute low back pain on the basis of this small study. Large-scale definitive trials are required to detect clinically significant differences.

QUESTIONS

1. Comment on the data given.
2. What information does $P < 0.05$ give the reader?
3. What extra information would you like to know before making a conclusion about the findings?

Your answers ....

48 HOURS' BED REST FOR BACK PAIN

Answers

Answer to question 1

Good points

Journal: Study published in a reputable journal.

Title: Relevant to general practice and common presenting complaint.

Author: Is the author a doctor, physiotherapist or a pure scientist? This would influence the way one would interpret the results.

Abstract: Easy to follow. A pilot study.

Aims: Clear.

Methods: A randomised, controlled, prospective trial; all these aspects make the study more robust.

Subjects
- A general practice setting; subjects are chosen in a way that allows some generalization to my current practice.
- A good age range: both elderly and young people get back pain.

Tests
- The Oswestry back pain questionnaire is a well-known and reliable test (and therefore easily repeatable). The Roland–Morris test is not so well-known and might not be so reliable.

Results: Apart from the Roland–Morris scores, at day 7 there was no statistical difference between the groups.

Conclusions: The conclusions drawn by the author were fair.

Bad points

Study: This was a pilot study with small numbers; therefore, firm conclusions cannot be made from the results. The abstract does not say whether or not it was a blind study.

Methods: Subjects
- Selection criteria and method of randomisation not mentioned.
- Patients came from West Midlands, which may represent an industrialized area with high numbers of social class 4 and 5. This may affect the degree to which the study can be generalized to one's own practice. The ethnic origin of the patients is also not mentioned. Ethnic origin is known to influence the way patients respond to illness.
- Gender not mentioned.
- The average age and age distribution may have given more information with such a wide age range.
- We are not told whether the patients are self-employed or not. This may affect whether or not they are willing to take time off work.

Design
- Patients with and without radiation of pain are all put together. This may lead to biased results if there is an uneven distribution in the two study groups. It may have been better to exclude those with radiation of their pain.
- The follow-up was only over the short term. A longer-term follow-up may have added more weight to the study.

Tests
The outcome measurements (i.e. SLR and lumbar flexion) may not be reliable indicators of recovery from back pain. They were measured after the episodes of pain but not before. We therefore have no information about each patient's baseline measurements. These are physical observations which are subject to observer error.

Results: The self-remedies were not defined and could affect the results.

Implications: The number of days off work was the same in the two groups. There was no difference between the two groups. Therefore, firm conclusions cannot be made regarding the treatment of low back pain.

Answer to question 2

The null hypothesis assumes that there is no difference in scores between those on bed rest and controls. $P < 0.05$ means that there is a less than 1 in 20 probability that this difference in Roland–Morris scores would occur by chance. This level of probability is chosen by convention to represent a statistically significant result. Statistical significance does not necessarily represent clinical significance.

Answer to question 3

- The results of a study repeated with larger numbers and a longer period of follow-up.
- Results of similar studies or meta-analyses would be helpful in making firm conclusions.
- Further studies that examined the psychological factors involved in getting people to lie flat for 48 hours.
- More information about the 'self-remedies'.

Comment

Positive points

- *Relevance:* Back pain is an important problem in general practice.
- *Randomised control trial:* Provides the strongest form of evidence.

Negative points

- *Contamination:* One cannot be sure whether the two groups were completely separate (i.e. that there was no mixing of treatments).
- *Low power:* The numbers in this study are too small to detect a statistically significant difference.
- *Consistency:* One would need to be sure that the different treatment centres gave the same advice to all patients.

In summary, a full-scale trial is required to draw a valid conclusion.

PREVALENCE OF ALCOHOL HISTORIES IN MEDICAL AND NURSING NOTES OF PATIENTS ADMITTED WITH SELF POISONING

Prevalence of alcohol histories in medical and nursing notes of patients admitted with self poisoning
R.M. Shepherd, M. London, T.H.S. Dent and G.J.M. Alexander
British Medical Journal (1995) **311**:847.
Reproduced with permission from the BMJ Publishing Group.

SUBJECTS, METHODS, AND RESULTS

As part of the evaluation of a training intervention to improve the management of excessive alcohol consumption among inpatients, we examined the medical and nursing notes and discharge summaries of consecutive patients admitted over 28 weeks to four general medical wards at a large teaching hospital. We recorded, among other items, the reason for admission and whether the notes and discharge summaries contained a quantified alcohol history, defined as a numerical record of consumption (including no consumption of alcohol). Knowledge of the reasons for admission could have biased the researcher's recording of the alcohol history, but this is unlikely, as the researcher examining the notes was not aware of the hypothesis that the two processes would be related. Patients were excluded if they could not speak English, were unconscious on admission, were less than 18 years old, were admitted as a day case, or were admitted on a second or subsequent occasion during the study. Men recorded as drinking more than 21 units a week and women recorded as drinking more than 14 units a week were regarded as excessive drinkers.

A total of 2680 patients were admitted during the study, 1955 (73%) of whose notes were examined and details of reason for admission and recorded alcohol history extracted. One hundred and forty five patients were admitted with self poisoning, 59 men and 86 women. Their ages ranged from 18 to 90 years (median 31). Fifty three of them had taken alcohol with their overdose of drugs. Only 37 had a quantitative alcohol history recorded in their medical notes, and 25 had a history recorded in their nursing notes, leaving 99 with no record in either set of notes. As shown in the table, patients admitted with self poisoning were less likely to have a quantitative alcohol history recorded than those admitted for other reasons. Only four of the 53 patients with self poisoning who took alcohol with their overdose had discharge summaries that mentioned their excessive drinking.

Numbers (percentages) of alcohol histories in medical and nursing notes of patients admitted with and without self poisoning

	Doctor's notes*		Nurse's notes†	
	Quantitative alcohol history	No quantitative alcohol history	Quantitative alcohol history	No quantitative alcohol history
Reason for admission:				
Self poisoning (n=145)	37 (26)	108 (74)	25 (17)	120 (83)
Not self poisoning (n=1810)	680 (38)	1130 (62)	459 (25)	1351 (75)

* $\chi^2 = 7.88$, $P = 0.005$ for proportion of notes with qualitative alcohol history, patients admitted with self poisoning v those admitted without self poisoning.
† $\chi^2 = 4.32$, $P = 0.04$ for proportion of notes with qualitative alcohol history, patients admitted with self poisoning v those admitted without self poisoning.

QUESTIONS

1. **Comment on the data given.**
2. **What actions might you take as a result of reading these data?**
3. **What conclusions can you make?**

Your answers ....

PREVALENCE OF ALCOHOL HISTORIES IN MEDICAL AND NURSING NOTES OF PATIENTS ADMITTED WITH SELF POISONING

Answers

Answer to question 1

Title: An evaluation of a 'training intervention'. Little relevance to general practice. However, may prompt general practitioners to ask their patients with drug problems about alcohol intake. May also prompt general practitioners to ask for alcohol histories on discharge summaries.

Methods: Setting
- Teaching hospital in Cambridge may not be generalizable to whole population.
- Doctors and nurses in teaching hospital may be more studious than those from a district general hospital or *vice versa*.

Exclusions
- The exclusion criteria are clearly set out. Only 73% of the notes were examined: what about the other notes? They may all have had alcohol histories recorded.
- Those that could not speak English, were under 18 years of age, or were unconscious are a very important group of people and likely to display a higher-than-average consumption of alcohol.

Subjects
- The subjects comprised 59 men and 86 women; the proportions are as might be expected. More women attempt parasuicide than men. Men are more likely to commit suicide.
- 18–90-year-old age group. This is a reasonable age range. Elderly people are often forgotten when it comes to excessive alcohol consumption. Not extending the age range to the under-18s may miss a significant group of problem drinkers.
- We are not told what level of medical staff recorded the histories: senior house officer, house officer, staff nurse, health care assistant?
- How reproducible is the study? Was a standardized protocol used? No details are given about the researchers. Were they trained to recognize medical short-hand (e.g. ETOH for alcohol)?

Design
- Observational study. No controls are used which may have strengthened the study.
- Length of stay is not recorded. It may be that those with a longer length of stay are more likely to have their alcohol history recorded.

Results: *P* values are given; however, confidence limits are not included. Doctors do better than nurses at recording alcohol histories. It may be that nurses do less recording because the alcohol history has already been recorded by the doctors. It is not clear whether this is the case from the data presented.

Answer to question 2

General practice
- As a GP I may do nothing as the results are not directly relevant to general practice.
- When referring patients as a GP I may include the alcohol history in my referral letters.
- I may ask for discharge summaries to contain the alcohol history and counsel excessive drinkers or refer them for specialist help.

Hospital
- Have pre-printed history sheets in notes which include details pertaining to the alcohol intake.
- Re-educate medical staff about history taking.
- Improve discharge summaries, so that the alcohol history can easily be recorded.
- Have an alcohol advisory service in the hospital to which patients can be referred.

General
- Audit or further studies should be carried out to gain more information on the subject.

Answer to question 3

There are few relevant conclusions to be made for general practice, except that doctors seem to be better at recording alcohol histories.

Comment
- Trained researchers and a standard protocol should be used to obtain **consistent measurements.**
- Hospital patients are the clinical **'tip of the iceberg'** (i.e. there will be more patients in the community who suffer from the disease).

In summary, this is an interesting study but its findings cannot be generalized to the whole population.

TRENDS IN PREVALENCE AND SEVERITY OF CHILDHOOD ASTHMA

Trends in prevalence and severity of childhood asthma
H.R.Anderson, B.K. Butland and D.P. Strachan
British Medical Journal (1994) **308**:1600
Reproduced with permission from the BMJ Publishing Group.

METHODS

In February 1978 and 1991 an identical one-page self completed questionnaire designed to screen for symptoms of asthma was distributed to the parents of all children in one school year (aged 7½ to 8½ years) attending all state and private schools in the borough. The questions were: has your child ever had asthma? And, if the answer to this question was no, has he or she ever had attacks of wheezing in the chest? Those who replied yes to either question were asked to record the number of attacks of asthma or wheezing illness over the past 12 months. In 1978 home interviews were sought from all parents reporting five or more attacks in the past year and a 52% sample of those reporting one to four attacks in the past year. Those patients reporting wheeze in the past 12 months but who provided no information on the frequency of attacks were treated for the purposes of sampling and subsequent analysis as if they had reported one to four attacks. In 1991 the parents of all wheezy children were included in the interview sample. The home interview covered a wide range of questions about the symptoms experienced and the impact of these on everyday life at home and at school; drug treatments and use of services; social, family, and economic factors; and possible causes and precipitating factors. These are described fully in reports of the 1978 survey.[9,10]

Tables I and II show the samples and response at both stages of the survey. The final analysis was based on 267 interviews for 1978 and 302 for 1991. Proportions of wheezy children with various symptoms were calculated and when appropriate extrapolated to provide estimates of population prevalence. Figures for 1978 were weighted to take account of differences in sampling fraction between frequent wheezers (100%) and infrequent wheezers (52%) (table II).

There were clearly differences in the two studies with respect to month of interview and lag time between screen and interview, which could bias the comparison (see table III). To adjust for these factors proportions among current wheezers were obtained by weighting the fitted values of logistic regression models containing month of interview as a 12 level factor, lag time as a linear trend, and a three level factor differentiating between 1991, 1978 infrequent wheeze, and 1978 frequent wheeze. Weights were used to take account of the differences in sampling fraction. Large sample 95% confidence intervals were calculated for the ratio of the adjusted proportions by using a method outlined by Flanders and Rhodes.[12]

Adjusted population prevalence ratios and their 95% confidence intervals were obtained by fitting Poisson regression models. As well as a term for year of study these models contained month of interview as a 12 level factor, lag time as a linear trend, and a two level factor for frequency of wheeze at screening. In fitting the Poisson regression models we assumed that among subjects with a disability or symptom of interest the probability of frequent wheeze was the same in 1978 as in 1991.

All models were fitted by using the LOGISTIC procedure of SAS.[13] When adjusted population prevalence estimates are quoted these are standardised to a November interview nine months after each screening survey.

[9] Anderson HR, Bailey PA, Cooper JS, Palmer JC, West S. Morbidity and school absence caused by asthma and wheezing illness. *Arch Dis Child* 1983; 83: 777–84.

[10] Anderson HR, Bailey PA, Cooper JS, Palmer JC, West S. Medical care of asthma and wheezing illness in children: a community survey. *J Epidemiol Community Health* 1983; 37: 180–6.

[11] Strachan DP, Anderson HR. Trends in hospital admission rates for asthma in children. *BMJ* 1992; 304: 873–5.

[12] Flanders WD, Rhodes PH. Large sample confidence intervals for regression standardised risks, risk ratios, and risk differences. *Journal of Chronic Disease* 1987; 40: 697–704.

[13] SAS Institute. SAS/STAT user's guide version 6. Vol 2. Cary, North Carolina: SAS Institute, 1989: 846.

[16] Anderson HR, Butland BK, Paine KM, Strachan DP. Trends in the medical care of asthma in childhood: Croydon 1978 and 1991. *Thorax* 1993; 48: 451.

TABLE I—*Samples and response in the two screening surveys*

Detail	Croydon 1978	Croydon 1991
Population targeted	4763	3786
Forms returned	4147	3070
Response rate	87%	81%
Wheeze in previous 12 months*	459	395

* Numbers differ slightly from those in earlier report[11] because of rediscovery of previously missing information on frequency of attacks in 1978 survey and addition of late responses in 1991 survey.

TABLE II—Samples and response in the two interview surveys

Detail	Croydon 1978*			Croydon 1991*		
	One to four attacks (including seven missing)	Five and more attacks	Total	One to four attacks (including six missing)	Five and more attacks	Total
Current wheezers identified at screen†	356	103	459	316	79	395
Sought for home interview	185‡	103	288	316	79	395
Interview obtained	178	95	273	253	66	319
Response rate		95%			81%	
After exclusions§	173	94	267	238	64	302

* Previous reports of interview data from 1978 survey[9,10,16] included some children from class above who were screened accidentally. For comparability with 1991 survey these older children have been excluded from this analysis.
† Numbers differ slightly from those in earlier report[11] because of rediscovery of previously missing information on frequency of attacks in 1978 survey and addition of late responses in 1991 survey.
‡ 52% Sample.
§ 1978 Study: five false positives, one unusable interview. 1991 Study: seven false positives, 10 stopped wheezing at interview (interviewed as former wheezers).

TABLE III—Proportions (percentages of those currently wheezy at screen) reported to have wheezed in month or 12 months before interview, according to season of interview and time lag between screen and interview

Detail		Season of interview*				Time lag in months					
	Study year	Spring	Summer	Autumn	Winter	1–4	5–7	8–10	11–13	>14	Total
No of subjects	1978	99	12	79	77	0	27	74	83	83	267
	1991	85	93	111	13	112	102	86	2	0	302
Percentage of total	1978	37	4	30	29	0	10	28	31	31	100
	1991	28	31	37	4	37	34	28	1	0	100
Percentage reported to have wheezed in month before interview	1978	13	40	43	42	†	41	39	40	12	31
	1991	59	66	57	67	62	57	64	†	†	61
Percentage reported to have wheezed in 12 months before interview	1978	89	80	90	86	†	91	88	89	85	88
	1991	95	100	92	100	96	98	92	†	†	96

* Spring = March, April, May; summer = June, July, August; autumn = September, October, November; winter = December, January, February.
† Estimates could not be calculated or were unreliable because of small number.

1. Comment on the information given.
2. Apart from any criticisms that you may have already made in answering question 1, what else would you like to know before making any conclusions about the trends in the prevalence of asthma in this age group?

Your answers ....

TRENDS IN PREVALENCE AND SEVERITY OF CHILDHOOD ASTHMA

Answers

Answer to question 1

Journal: This study is published in a reputable journal, which will positively influence the way I react to the conclusions I make about the study.

Title: Asthma is a subject which is relevant to general practice. The trends in the prevalence of asthma have been said to be increasing and hence the findings of this study will be of particular interest.

Author: The author is a professor of Public Health and one would therefore expect the paper to be of a reasonably high standard.

Methods: This is a cross-sectional survey, which is a standard way to assess prevalence.

The questionnaire
- The reproducibility of the study will be influenced by the validity (measures what it is supposed to) of the questionnaire. This information is not available to us.
- The questionnaire is a reasonable way to assess the prevalence of asthma, although a more specific way to look at asthma prevalence would be to assess airway responsiveness. It is known that the management of asthma has improved over the years so that the number of wheezy attacks per year can be reduced. This may skew the results if prevalence is assessed by looking at symptoms alone.
- A one-page questionnaire is a good idea. It is known that people are more likely to complete a one-page questionnaire than a questionnaire with several pages.
- A response rate of over 75% allows good comparisons to be made between the two years of the survey. However, the response rate after the exclusions were made is not given.
- The questions are easy to understand.
- The parents are asked to remember how many attacks of asthma or wheeze had occurred in the last 12 months. This may be unreliable because it relies on memory.

Interviews
- In 1978, interviews were conducted on those with severe asthma. In 1991, interviews were conducted on all those with wheezy symptoms. The reason for this inconsistency is not given.
- We are not told why a 52% sample of the group having 1–4 attacks per year were selected for interview.
- We are not told whether the same interview was used in both 1978 and 1991. It is very unlikely that this is the case. Therefore, there is likely to be some element of inconsistency in the interviewing techniques and styles between the two years. This element of bias may have been lessened if the interviewers were trained in a formalised way but this information is not included.
- Although an attempt has been made to correct for the lag time between screen and interview, and the month of interview, this may still have skewed the results.

Subjects
- The subjects are from Croydon but we are not given the general characteristics or demographics (e.g. social class, whether subjects smoke or not) of this population. It is therefore difficult to assess whether this population is typical of the whole population of the UK. It may therefore be difficult to generalize the results.
- There is no clear definition of asthma and wheeze. Parents may mistake other viral illness such as croup for asthma; this may influence the prevalence results, especially if there was an epidemic of such an illness in one of the years of survey.
- We are not told why only 3786 people were targeted in 1991 while 1000 people more were targeted in 1978. Was it an attempt to cut the costs of the study? If so, what other cost-cutting measurements were used and could they affect our interpretation of the results?
- No information is given about the drop-outs.
- The increase in prevalence seen in 1991 may be due to increased awareness rather than a true increase in asthma.

Tables
- The tables are quite straightforward except that 'false positives' are not explained.

Statistics
- The methods appear complex so it is difficult to comment.

Answer to question 2

- The results of other studies would be useful, particularly those which looked at specific measurements of asthma, such as hospital admissions and bronchial hyperresponsiveness tests.

- Knowledge of other environmental factors occurring at the time of the study, such as local pollution or viral epidemics, would be useful.

Comment

Cross-sectional study: The limitations of a cross-sectional study are mentioned elsewhere.

Case definition: A good definition of asthma is required.

Secular trends are changes in prevalence over time. They can be attributed to a number of factors including artefacts, increased awareness and access to services.

Verification: It is important to use other sources of data to verify this finding.

In summary, this is an interesting study. The findings are relevant to general practice but need to be supported by other studies.

SELECTIVE SEROTONIN RE-UPTAKE INHIBITORS FOR DEPRESSION (SSRIs)

Selective serotonin re-uptake inhibitors for depression
Drug and Therapeutics Bulletin (1993) **31**: 51–58
published by Consumers' Association, 2 Marylebone Road, London NW1 4DF

CLINICAL EFFECTIVENESS

The tricyclic antidepressants, at doses of 125–150 mg per day or greater, are effective in the treatment of moderate to severe depression, and these drugs are the standard with which SSRIs must be compared.

SSRIs have been evaluated against tricyclic and 'related' antidepressants (eg mianserin, maprotiline, trazadone) in a meta-analysis of randomised trials involving hospital inpatients, outpatients and patients in general practice. All had major depression, as judged by the Hamilton score. The median length of follow up was 6 weeks. Analysis of the 20 trials (1800 patients) giving sufficient data for pooling showed that SSRIs and tricyclic and related antidepressants were of equal efficacy. About a third of patients receiving SSRIs and a third of those receiving tricyclic and related antidepressants dropped out of treatment: 15% and 19%, respectively, withdrew because of side effects and 7% from each group withdrew because they found the treatment ineffective.

Approximate prices of 6 months' treatment at BNF recommended doses

Antidepressant	Daily dose	Cost
Selective serotonin re-uptake inhibitors		
Fluoxetine	20 mg	£116
Fluvoxamine	100–200 mg	£140–280
Paroxetine	20 mg	£190
Sertraline	50–100 mg	£160–240
Tricyclic antidepressants		
Amitryptyline	50–100 mg	£3–6
Clomipramine	50–100 mg	£19–38
Dothiepin	75–150 mg	£21–42
Imipramine	150–200 mg	£6–8
Lofepramine	140–210 mg	£62–92

QUESTIONS

1. Comment on the data given in the above text on 'clinical effectiveness'. What are the implications of such information?
2. What additional information would you like to know before making your own conclusions about the clinical effectiveness of SSRIs over tricyclic antidepressants (TCAs)?
3. Given the information in the above table on cost, how do you decide which drug to prescribe?
4. What further information would you require to appraise this meta-analysis?

Your answers ....

SELECTIVE SEROTONIN RE-UPTAKE INHIBITORS FOR DEPRESSION (SSRIs)

Answers

Answer to question 1

Good points

- *Drug and Therapeutics Bulletin* is a reputable journal; its conclusions are more likely to be generally accepted.
- Relevant to general practice. SSRIs are seen as a major rival to TCAs; it is important to make informed decisions about prescribing.
- Large number of patients surveyed.
- All trials were randomised.
- Using a meta-analysis in this situation is probably a good idea, because it is difficult to collect large numbers of depressed patients.
- Hamilton rating is a validated method of scoring the severity of depression.

Bad points

- Patients are collected from different sources (inpatients, outpatients and general practice). Therefore, the results may not be directly applicable to general practice.
- No statistical evidence is presented.
- Meta-analyses can be misleading. A critical appraisal of the meta-analysis is also required.
- Depressive illness can go on for longer than 6 weeks. A longer period of follow-up would have been more appropriate.
- 'Efficacy' is not defined. What outcome measurements are used to define efficacy?
- Drop-outs are mentioned but the side-effects experienced by these subjects is not mentioned. Suicides and parasuicides are not mentioned. Confounding factors are also not mentioned.

Implications

There seems to be no real incentive to prescribe SSRIs over the older TCAs. However, SSRIs are an alternative to TCAs, if required.

Answer to question 2

Study design
- Drop-outs. Over 70% of the drop-outs are not accounted for. Why did they drop out of the study? Will this affect my clinical decision-making?
- Statistical tests should be provided, such as confidence intervals and P values.
- What are the long-term effects of SSRIs?
- What is the long-term outcome of using SSRIs compared with TCAs?
- Confounding factors, such as premorbid personality, alcohol use or other significant past medical history, should be taken into account.

The drug
- Side-effect profile
- Contraindications
- How safe is an overdose?

Results of other studies
Studies relevant to general practice are preferable.

Answer to question 3

Cost alone should not dictate whether or not a drug is prescribed. The following should be taken into account as well:

Patient considerations
- Dosage regime; for example, once a day will be better tolerated than multiple daily doses.
- Patient preference (what have they tried in the past).
- Additional benefits of the drug (such as sleep or reduction in anxiety).
- Contraindications (such as prostate disease and the administration of TCAs).

Drug considerations
- Side-effect profile in different age groups.
- Safety of overdose.
- How long does it take for the drug to work?

Practice considerations
- What are the local guidelines for the prescription of antidepressants?
- Need to compare the cost of equivalent doses of different antidepressants.

Answer to question 4

To include
- Search methods including non-English databases and unpublished research.
- Explicit inclusion criteria of high quality studies.
- Inclusion of studies which are broadly similar in populations and design.
- Table displaying the individual studies.
- Plot of the trials.
- Statistical test of heterogeneity.
- Overall pooled result including confidence intervals.

DATA INTERPRETATION

- These questions are not as difficult as the critical appraisal questions but it is important that you get a feel for the technique involved and learn to write clear and concise answers.

- The answers given are 'consensus' answers.

- Give yourselves 15 minutes for each question.

OUTPATIENTS' WAITING TIMES

The table shows the outpatient waiting times for two hospitals in your practice area.

Outpatients' waiting times for breast surgery

Hospital	Doctor	Waiting time
A	Q	14 weeks (urgent appointment: 3 weeks)
	P	4 weeks
B (a one-stop breast clinic)	All	3 weeks (urgent appointment: immediately)

QUESTIONS

1. Comment on the difference between the two hospitals. What factors may cause such a discrepancy in waiting times?
2. How do you decide which hospital to send your patient to?

Your answers ....

OUTPATIENTS' WAITING TIMES

Answers

Answer to question 1

Hospital A has much longer waiting times than hospital B. There is a discrepancy between doctors and within hospital A. The waiting time for urgent appointments to see Doctor P is not mentioned. We are not told whether the hospitals are private or NHS hospitals. It is difficult to compare hospital A with hospital B because one appears to be a rapid access clinic and the other an ordinary outpatient clinic.

Hospital A
- Three weeks is a long time to wait for an urgent appointment.
- Hospital A may be closer to the practice than hospital B.
- Hospital A may have an interest in a speciality other than breast surgery.
- Patients may prefer hospital A to hospital B.
- May be underfunded or understaffed.
- May be under poor management.

Hospital B (one-stop breast clinic)
- The number of doctors serving this clinic is not mentioned.
- The hospital may have deliberately set about trying to get referrals from local GPs by improving their service and having designated breast clinics every day.
- They may have such a short wait because the patients see junior doctors rather than consultants.
- They may be more efficient at managing breast cases because of agreed protocols that are followed by all staff.
- The short wait may also be because the clinic or hospital is new and therefore has few patients.

Doctor Q
- May be very popular with patients or GPs.
- May be part-time.
- May be poorly organized.
- May have been off sick.
- May be a woman and therefore more popular with women patients.
- May have a lot of follow-up appointments.

Doctor P

- May be a new doctor.
- May not be well respected.
- May be working in breast surgery only and therefore has more appointments.

Answer to question 2

- Knowledge of the consultants, their reputation, skill and experience.
- Waiting time is very important with respect to the anxiety of the patient and of her family.
- Distance to travel to the hospital and ease of access on public transport and by car.
- Cost to practice (if fundholding) or health authority.
- Patient preference for hospital or consultant and also for private or NHS hospital.
- Service offered by the hospital, which includes the availability of hospital doctors to discuss problems, quality of follow-up, quality of discharge summaries, etc..
- The perceived urgency of the clinical condition.
- Published audit data from breast clinic or trust.

PRESCRIBING DATA 1

Prescribing data can be depicted in graphical form. The graphs below represent two practices, A and B, taken from areas which have the same postcode. Assume that both are three-partner practices with the same number of patients.

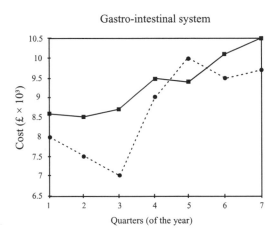

Gastro-intestinal system

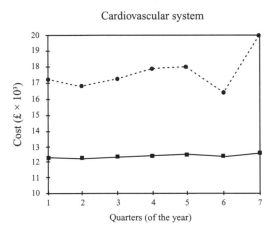

Cardiovascular system

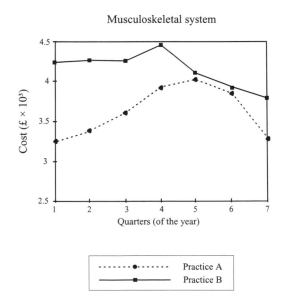

Musculoskeletal system

Practice A
Practice B

QUESTIONS

1. (a) For each graph, give reasons for the difference between the prescribing costs for practices A and B. Also comment on the individual variations in the prescribing costs.

   (b) What additional information might you need to make sense of the differences?

2. (a) For practice A, how might you investigate the high prescribing costs for cardiovascular drugs?

   (b) If you found the costs to be inappropriately high, what techniques could be used to modify the prescribing behaviour of Practice A?

Your answers . . . .

PRESCRIBING DATA 1

Answers

Answer to question 1(a)

Gastro-intestinal system

Prescribing in practice A tends to be slightly less than in practice B. Possible reasons include:

- Shorter waiting list for gastro-intestinal endoscopy or 'open access' available in practice A, meaning that the patient spends less time on drugs before a definite diagnosis is made or treatment occurs.
- Practices A and B may have completely different populations of patients, even if they are within the same postcode. Practice B may have more socially deprived patients, with a higher incidence of smoking, stress, or more elderly patients.
- Practice A may be more efficient at generic prescribing.
- Practice A may have been under-diagnosing.
- Practice B may have been over-diagnosing.
- Practice A may have more private patients or use more alternative therapies.

There is an increase in prescribing after the third quarter for practice A. Possible reasons include:

- A new partner could have joined the practice who may be accustomed to prescribing more expensive drugs.
- Practice A may have a general increase in gastro-intestinal problems.
- Practice A may have improved their diagnosis and treatment of gastro-intestinal problems.
- A drug representative may have influenced prescribing.
- An increase in patient awareness of symptoms may have occurred after an education campaign in the media or in the practice.

Cardiovascular system

Practice A has much higher prescribing costs than practice B. Possible reasons include:

Wrong data.

Practice A:
- Over-diagnosing or incorrect diagnosis.

- Brand-name prescribing.
- Premature treatment of high blood pressure.
- Differing populations. Afro-Caribbeans tend to respond better to third or fourth line antihypertensives rather than to the cheaper first or second line drugs. There may be a lot of Asian diabetics with cardiovascular disease at this practice.
- Drug representative influencing prescribing.
- A partner with a special interest in the cardiovascular system.
- There may be a few patients on very expensive drugs prescribed by the hospital consultant.

Practice B:
- Under-diagnosing.
- Using alternative therapies.
- Lots of private patients, whose private prescriptions may not appear in this data.

Musculoskeletal system
Practice A tends to have lower prescribing costs than Practice B. Possible reasons include:

Practice A:
- Under-diagnosing.
- Quick access to physiotherapy or alternative practitioners such as acupuncturists or chiropractors.
- The peaks in the 5th and 7th quarters may have occurred due to:
  (a) A locum who was unaware of practice facilities.
  (b) A hospital prescribing for patients discharged from hospital.
  (c) The influence of a drug representative.
- The decline in prescribing costs after the 7th quarter may be secondary to an education initiative.

Practice B:
The on-going general decrease in prescribing costs may be secondary to:

- On-going audit and review of prescribing.
- The steeper decrease around the 4th quarter may be a result of employing a new partner interested in non-drug therapies or the introduction of physiotherapy.

Answer to question 1(b)

- Age: sex ratio of the two practices.
- Special interests of the partners.
- In-house facilities.
- Social class structure of both practices.
- Proportion of private patients or private prescriptions in each practice.

Answer to question 2(a)

- Look at the prescribing costs for each individual partner.
- Look at the proportion of generic prescribing.
- Review the diagnoses on all the patients taking cardiovascular drugs.
- Compare the prescribing with a practice which has been matched for age, sex, social class, etc. [e.g. use the Prescription Pricing Authority (PPA) data].
- Look at the appropriateness of prescribing by assessing the outcome of the disease (e.g. angina, hypertension).
- Ask for help from outside agencies (e.g. PPA, Local Medical Advisor).

Answer to question 2(b)

- Perform regular audits using protocols acceptable to the partners.
- Use computers which convert brand names to generics and which inform the prescriber of the cost of the drug.
- Use all the partners, together with the pharmacist or medical advisor, to develop a practice formulary.

PRESCRIBING DATA 2

Prescribing data can be depicted in terms of the 'number of items prescribed' and the 'average cost per item'.

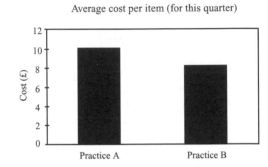

Number of items prescribed

Average cost per item (for this quarter)

QUESTIONS

1. What is an item?
2. What information can be derived from 'the number of items prescribed' and the 'average cost per item'?
3. The charts clearly show that the 'number of items prescribed' for practice A is less than that for practice B. However, the 'average cost per item' in practice A is higher than that in practice B. How do you explain this difference?
4. List the positive and negative points about the information derived from the prescribing data.

Your answers ....

PRESCRIBING DATA 2

Answers

Answer to question 1

An item is a prescribed drug or article.

Answer to question 2

- The 'number of items prescribed' is a means of assessing the total volume of a drug prescribed. However, it gives no information about the quantity of a drug present in the prescription (i.e. the number of tablets per item or ml of fluid per item).
- The 'average cost per item' together with the 'number of items prescribed', sometimes known as prescribing variables, have been found to correlate with unemployment rates and other measures of deprivation. A high number of items with a low cost per item has been correlated with increased levels of deprivation.

Answer to question 3

- Practice A may represent a practice situated in a relatively affluent area. In this situation, one might expect the patients to visit their GP relatively infrequently but be prescribed more expensive drugs. The reverse might be true for practice B, the patients of which might be expected to make frequent trips to their GP for relatively minor complaints, requiring less expensive drugs.
- Practice A may have a few of its patients on very expensive drugs, such as infertility drugs or chemotherapy drugs.
- The lower 'average cost per item' in practice B could represent a proportion of generic prescribing.
- The higher 'average cost per item' in practice A could represent a larger quantity of drug in each item compared with practice B.

Answer to question 4

Positive points
- Encourages awareness of finances.
- Encourages production of practice formulary.
- Encourages use of audit.

Negative point
- Emphasis on cost rather than quality of care.

GUIDELINES

- Guidelines are part of our everyday practice in primary care. They provide a set of recommendations for the appropriate management of a particular condition and should be based on the best available evidence.

- Answer questions 1–3 in 15 minutes.

GUIDELINES

QUESTIONS

1. List the processes involved in guideline formation.
2. List the important points involved in the critical appraisal of guidelines.
3. List the positive and negative points regarding the use and implementation of guidelines.

Your answers ....

GUIDELINES

Answer to question 1

- Assign guideline development group.
- Identify key question/s.
- Perform a systematic search for evidence.
- Analyse evidence and compile an evidence table for each key question.
- Construct recommendations based on the evidence.
- Compile a draft set of guidelines and send them for external review.
- Publish guidelines.
- Make plans for review/update of guidelines.

It must be pointed out that not just anyone can sit down and write a guideline. Guideline development groups are made up of people who have experience and expertise in the topic in question. They will include health professionals and patients and technical experts.

Answer to question 2

(1) Assemble 2–4 appraisers.
(2) Appraise the following 6 domains:
- Scope and purpose.
- Stakeholder involvement.
- Rigour of development.
- Clarity of presentation.
- Applicability.
- Editorial independence.

The Appraisal of Guidelines for Research and Evaluation (AGREE) collaboration (September 2001) has formulated an instrument to aid in the critical appraisal of guidelines. The aim of the instrument is to identify potential biases in the development of the guideline and to assess whether or not the recommendations made in the guideline are internally and externally valid as well as feasible in practice.

The instrument consists of the 6 domains mentioned above. Each domain contains several items which are scored on a 4-point scale which ranges from 4—'strongly agree' to 1—'strongly disagree'. In order to increase the reliability of the instrument, it is suggested that any guideline is assessed by at least 2 but preferably 4 appraisers.

Scope and development

The guideline should clearly describe the following:

- Objectives of the guideline including the health benefits.
- The clinical question/s to be covered.
- The patients to whom the guideline applies.

Stakeholder involvement

Those involved in developing the guideline should include the appropriate professional groups. The views of patients should be sought. The target users should be clearly defined and this group should also have been piloted.

Rigour of development

- A systematic approach should have been used to search for evidence.
- Criteria for selecting evidence should be clearly defined.
- Methods used to formulate recommendations should be clear.
- Benefits and harms should have been considered in making the recommendations.
- There should be a clear link between recommendations and the evidence used.
- The guideline should be reviewed externally.
- There should be clear procedures for updating the guideline.

Clarity and presentation

- The recommendations of the guideline should be clearly presented and unambiguous.
- The various options for management should be clear.
- Any key recommendations should be clearly identified.
- Tools for easy use of the instrument should be provided alongside the guideline e.g. leaflets, computer support.

Applicability

The cost and organisational implications of using the guideline should have been discussed. Data that aid in audit of the guideline should be included e.g. specific targets for blood pressure or blood glucose control.

Editorial independence

The guideline should be editorially independent from the funding body and any conflicts of interest should be clearly defined.

Overall assessment

Finally the appraiser is asked whether or not he/she would recommend the use of the guideline. The appraiser is asked to tick one of 4 boxes (strongly recommend, recommend, would not recommend, unsure).

Answer to question 3

Positive points

Guidelines improve the process of care, e.g.

- They aid in the development of standards of care.
- They can be used in education and training.
- They may help patients to make informed choices.
- They may help to improve communication between health professionals.

Guidelines may also improve the outcome of care.

Negative points

- Guidelines do not replace knowledge and skills.
- They may be biased, e.g. in favour of economically more favourable treatments.
- Different organisations use different systems for developing and grading guideline recommendations.
- They are only good if they are used.
- They are only good if they are updated regularly.
- Guideline recommendations identify those issues which are supported by the strongest evidence. However, it may be more important to look at the issue that is likely to produce the greatest clinical impact.
- Qualitative studies may provide valuable information but are not incorporated into the guideline development process.

The international **GRADE** (Grades of Recommendation, Assessment, Development and Evaluation) project has identified several areas of weakness of current systems and has made recommendations for change. These include assessing the quality, not just of the overall study but also as it relates to the key question/outcome. Each question/outcome should be given a predefined level of importance. As well as benefits of treatments, harms should also be assessed. The cost implications should also be incorporated into the guideline recommendations.

Levels of evidence

Once a systematic search for evidence has been performed, it is the job of the guideline development group to analyse the evidence and assign a 'level of evidence' to each study. The assigned level will depend on the type and quality of the study. This evidence can then be used to formulate a set of recommendations (graded from A to D).

You will find several different systems in operation. The Scottish Intercollegiate Guideline Network (SIGN) and the National Institute for Clinical Excellence (NICE) use similar systems. SIGN and NICE have meta-analyses as level 1 evidence and expert opinion as level 4 evidence. They then divide level 1 and 2 (systematic reviews, cohort and case control studies) according to quality (++, + or –).

Grades of recommendation

The translation of evidence into a recommendation is straightforward if the evidence is high quality and is directly applicable to the key question. In this situation level 1 evidence may directly result in a grade A recommendation. However, this is often not the case. The evidence may be poor or may not directly relate to the key question. For example, the question may relate to the management of diabetes in children and the evidence may pertain to the management of diabetes in adults. In this situation an extrapolation of evidence may be necessary.

Grading systems for recommendations vary but in general, grade A recommendations are based on level 1 evidence. A grade D recommendation will be based on level 4 evidence or extrapolated evidence from studies higher up in the hierarchy.

It is interesting to note that 'Clinical Evidence' does not use hierarchy levels. Instead it describes the study in question.

PART II

- Risk and NNT
- Screening

RISK AND NNT

- Risk is a measure of the probability (or the chance) of something happening.
- Risk factors are associated with an increased chance of developing a given disease.
- Absolute, relative and attributable risks are covered in the first section.
- The 'numbers needed to treat' or NNT is a simpler method of conveying the risks and benefits of interventions. For those of us that find the concept of 'risk' difficult to grasp, NNT should prove a more useful aid to clinical decision-making.

INFORMATION ON RISK

Risk is a measure of the probability (or the chance) of something happening.

Absolute risk, relative risk and attributable risk can be calculated using data from cohort studies. Because case-control studies are not representative of the general population, absolute risk, relative risk and attributable risk cannot be calculated directly using data from these studies. The odds ratio can be calculated using data from case-control studies and is an estimate of the relative risk.

The absolute risk is equivalent to the background incidence of disease in the general population. Relative risk and attributable risk are measures of association.

- Relative risk gives an indication of the magnitude of the association between 'exposure' (or presence of a risk factor) and outcome (or for example development of the disease). Attributable risk is the excess risk or outcome that can be attributed to a given exposure.
- The higher the relative risk, the higher the likelihood that the factor in question is associated with the disease.

For both case-control and cohort studies, the same 2×2 table is used to calculate relative and attributable risk.

		Disease (or outcome)		
		Present	Absent	
Exposure	Present	A	B	(A + B)
	Absent	C	D	(C + D)
		(A + C)	(B + D)	(A + B + C + D)

COHORT STUDIES

For a cohort study, we start with (A+B) (exposed group) and (C+D) (non-exposed group). The subjects are then followed-up so that the rate of new disease occurrence (incidence) can be calculated.

Relative risk

The disease rate in the exposed group is compared with the disease rate in the non-exposed group. In other words, the disease rate in the exposed group is divided by the disease rate in the non-exposed group:

$$\text{Relative risk} = \frac{A}{(A+B)} \div \frac{C}{(C+D)} = \frac{A\times(C+D)}{C\times(A+B)}$$

It is important to remember that the relative risk does not give an indication of the probability of developing the disease. For example, the relative risk of developing a venous thromboembolism when using the oral contraceptive pill may be high. But, if venous thromboembolism is rare, the benefits of pill use may outweigh the risks.

Attributable risk

The attributable risk is the excess risk (or outcome) that can be attributed to a given exposure and therefore removes the background risk in the general population. It is a much more useful tool for decision-making than the relative risk but can only be calculated directly from data using cohort studies; that is, when the incidence of the disease can be calculated. The relative risk of two diseases may be the same but if one of the diseases is rarer than the other, the attributable risk for the rarer disease will be less. Another way of looking at it is that attributable risk is dependent on the prevalence of the disease in the population.

The attributable risk is calculated by subtracting the disease rate in the non-exposed group from the disease rate in the exposed group:

$$\text{Attributable risk} = \frac{A}{(A+B)} - \frac{C}{(C+D)}$$

CASE-CONTROL STUDIES

In a case-control study, the total number of subjects with the disease (A+C) are known. The total number of controls (B+D) are also known. The number of subjects exposed are counted, so that the values A and B can be added to the 2 × 2 table. The number of those who are not exposed or who do not have the potential risk factor are counted, so that the value (C+D) can be added to the table. Exposure rates for the cases and controls can then be worked out:

$$\text{Exposure rate for cases} = \frac{A}{(A+C)}$$

$$\text{Exposure rate for controls} = \frac{B}{(B+D)}$$

ODDS RATIO (CASE-CONTROL STUDIES)

As already mentioned, the true relative risk cannot be calculated using data from case-control studies. It can, however, be estimated. This estimate is called the odds ratio. In actual fact, many studies will still call it the relative risk. We know that the equation for the true relative risk is given by:

$$\text{Relative risk} = \frac{A \times (C+D)}{C \times (A+B)}$$

If the incidence of the disease is small (< 5%) and the control group are representative of the general population, then:

- C will be much smaller than D.

This means that:

- (A+B) will be a similar number (approximate) to B and
- (C+D) will be a similar number (approximate) to D.

Hence, $\dfrac{A \times (C+D)}{C \times (A+B)}$ will approximate to $\dfrac{(A \times D)}{(C \times B)}$

WORKED EXAMPLE OF RISK QUESTION

Oral contraception and risk of a cerebral thromboembolic attack: results of a case-control study.
Øjvind Lidegaard
British Medical Journal (1993) **306**, 956–963
Reproduced with permission from the BMJ Publishing Group.

TABLE II—*Included and excluded cases and controls and their respective use of oral contraceptives*

	No (%)	% Use of oral contraceptives (n)
Cases		
Submitted questionnaires		692
Returned questionnaires		590 (85.3)
Refusals	15	
Earlier cerebral thromboembolic attack (before 1980)	9	
Wrong diagnosis*	44	
Unreliable diagnosis†	25	
Reliable diagnosis		497	32.6 (161/494)
Confounder control		174
Previous thromboembolic disease	31		16.1 (5/31)
Pregnancy	13		–
Predisposition‡:		
Hypertension (treated)	68		26.5 (18/68)
Migraine (more than once a month)	49		30.6 (15/49)
Other conditions‖	35		28.6 (10/35)
Non-predisposed women with cerebral thromboembolic attacks¶		323	36.3 (116/320)
Occlusion of precerebral artery (ICD 432)	10		30.0 (3/10)
Cerebral thrombosis (ICD 433)	114		38.9 (44/113)
Cerebral embolism (ICD 434)	15		53.3 (8/15)
Transient cerebral ischaemia (ICD 435)	86		30.2 (26/86)
Cerebral haemorrhage (ICD 436)	98		36.5 (35/96)
Controls		
Submitted questionnaires		1584
Returned questionnaires		1396 (88.1)
Refusals, moved, retarded	8	
Uncompleted questionnaires	18	
Completed questionnaires		1370	15.2 (208/1369)
Confounder control		172
Previous thromboembolic disease	17		5.9 (1/17)
Pregnancy	31		‡
Predisposition‡		
Hypertension (treated)	56		7.1 (4/56)
Migraine (more than once a month)	62		17.7 (11/62)
Other conditions‖	12		8.3 (1/12)
Non-predisposed controls¶		1198	16.0 (191/1197)

* Multiple sclerosis, migraine, brain tumour.
† If patient denied having had a cerebral thromboembolic attack or stated that it occurred more than one year after the time recorded in the National Patient Register.
‡ As far as predisposition was expected to influence the use of oral contraceptives. Including 15 with migraine.
‖ Cases/controls: connective tissue disease 11/8, coagulopathy 2/0, hyperlipidaemia 4/0, tetraplegia 1/0, psychosis 2/1, severe brain damage 2/1, brain abscess 1/0, heart disease 12/1, brain aneurysm 0/1.
¶ 'Non-predisposed' refers to women free of confounding predisposing diseases.

QUESTIONS

1. Using the table given, work out the odds ratio of developing cerebral thromboembolism among users compared with non-users of the oral contraceptive pill. Draw a 2 × 2 table and show how you arrive at your final answer. (NB: because the numbers used in this example are actual numbers, you will need to use a calculator. In the exam, the numbers are usually worked out so that calculators are not required).
2. How would you explain the significance of this number to your patient?

Your answers ....

WORKED EXAMPLE OF RISK QUESTION

Answers

Answer to question 1

		(Disease) Cerebral thromboembolism	
		Present	**Absent**
Pill use (Exposure)	**Present**	A = 116	B = 191
	Absent	C = 204	D = 1006
		320 (A+C)	1197 (B+D)

According to the data given, after confounding factors are taken into account, 116 out of 320 women with cerebral thromboembolism were using the pill. C can thus be calculated as 320 minus 116. For the controls, after confounding variables are taken into consideration, 191 out of 1197 controls were using the pill. D can thus be calculated as 1197 minus 191.

$$\text{Odds Ratio} = \frac{(A \times D)}{(C \times B)} = \frac{116 \times 1006}{204 \times 191} = \frac{116696}{38964} = 3$$

The odds ratio of developing cerebral thromboembolism in pill users is 3. This means that pill users are three times more likely than non-pill users to develop cerebral thromboembolism.

Answer to question 2

Understanding risk is difficult. It would be important to avoid alarming the patient (by saying that there is a 300% increase in risk). Cerebral thromboembolism in younger women is fairly rare. It would be best to talk about the attributable risk of the pill. For example, suppose that in a population of 10 000 healthy women under 45 years of age, who were not pill users, only one suffers cerebral thromboembolism in a year. If the whole of this population did use the oral contraceptive pill, the number would be three per year.

QUESTIONS ON RISK

QUESTIONS

1. In a cohort study, a group of individuals is classified according to the presence or absence of a measured exposure. They are then followed-up over a period of time to measure the disease rates in exposed and non-exposed groups. From the diagram below, devise a 2 × 2 table that you could use to calculate the relative risk of disease in exposed compared with non-exposed individuals.

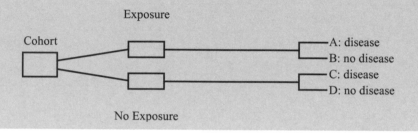

Your answer ....

2. If the above study gave a relative risk of 1.0, how would you interpret the effect of the exposure?

Your answer ....

3. The Committee on Safety of Medicines (CSM) released data from studies assessing the risks of thromboembolism associated with the use of HRT [Committee on Safety of Medicines/Medicines Control Agency. *Current Problems in Pharmacovigilance* (1996) 22:9]. The following results are taken from the patient information sheet:

Chances of a blood clot in patients:

Not taking HRT – 1 in 10 000

Taking HRT – 3 in 10 000

(a) What is the absolute risk (incidence) of thrombosis in the general female population?

(b) What is the relative risk of thrombosis in those taking HRT compared with non-users?

(c) What is the attributable risk of thrombosis in HRT users compared with the rest of the population?

Your answer ....

4. One of the original CSM studies used hospital-based cases and controls. Outline the reasons why it is reasonable to use the odds ratio calculated from this case-control study as an approximation to the relative risk of thrombosis.

Your answer ....

5. Prior to recent publications, HRT was thought to have a beneficial effect in reducing the risk of ischaemic heart disease by about 40%. It was also thought to be associated with a slight increase in the risk of breast cancer after 10 years of up to 30%.
(a) Given those figures, work out the relative risk of ischaemic heart disease in HRT users compared with non-users?
(b) Work out the relative risk of breast cancer in HRT users compared with non-users?

Your answer ....

QUESTIONS ON RISK

Answers

Answer to question 1

		Disease (or outcome)		
		Yes	No	
Exposure	Yes	A	B	(A + B)
	No	C	D	(C + D)
		(A + C)	(B + D)	(A + B + C + D)

The relative risk is the incidence of disease in the exposed population divided by the incidence in the non-exposed population:

$$\frac{A}{(A+B)} \div \frac{C}{(C+D)}$$

Answer to question 2

The exposure is not associated with an increased or decreased risk of the disease in this study. It has no effect on the disease.

Answer to question 3

(a)   1 in 10 000

		Disease (thrombosis)		
		Yes	No	
HRT use	Yes	3	99 997	10 000
	No	1	99 999	10 000

(b) Relative risk is the incidence of disease in the exposed population divided by the incidence in the non-exposed population:

$$\frac{3}{10\ 000} \div \frac{1}{10\ 000} = 3$$

(c) Attributable risk is the incidence in the exposed population minus the incidence in the non-exposed population:

$$\frac{3}{10\ 000} - \frac{1}{10\ 000} = \frac{2}{10\ 000} = 0.0002$$

Answer to question 4

See p. 89 (Case-control studies).

Answer to question 5

(a) Relative risk is the ratio of disease incidence in the exposed population to that in the non-exposed population. In this case, the population is exposed to HRT.
If the risk is 1 in the non-exposed population, reducing this risk by 40% leads to a risk in the exposed population of:
$1 - (40\% \text{ of } 1) = 0.6$

(b) If we take the risk in the non-exposed population as 1, increasing this by 30% leads to a risk in the exposed population of:
$1 + (30\% \text{ of } 1) = 1.3$

NUMBERS NEEDED TO TREAT (NNT)

The numbers needed to treat (NNT) is another method of communicating risks and benefits. For intervention trials it is defined simply as:

> The number of individuals who 'on average' would need to be treated to achieve one desired outcome or event.

It is more useful in decision-making than relative risks and attributable risks. It gives you some idea of whether a treatment is worth performing in your population.

> It is derived from the reciprocal of the reduction in absolute risk (absolute risk reduction or ARR) as a percentage term
>
> $$\frac{1}{ARR\ \%}$$

The absolute risk reduction (ARR) is the difference between the event rate in treated individuals and controls for a therapeutic trial (see below).

ARR = (proportion of the treated group with the desired outcome) – (proportion of controls with the desired outcome)

ARR% = (% of the treated group with the desired outcome) – (% of controls with the desired outcome)

This means that the NNT is dependent on the prevalence of a given disorder. Those disorders which are common (high absolute risk or incidence), such as heart disease, would have a low NNT to prevent one death. Rare disorders would mean that a large number of patients need to be treated to prevent a death.

Example

A study of nicotine replacement to aid smoking cessation was conducted in 200 patients. After 3 months, 36 out of 200 patients in the treatment group had stopped smoking; 22 out of 200 people had stopped smoking in the control group.

- The desired outcome here is giving up smoking.
- The percentage giving up smoking in the treatment group is 18%.
- The percentage giving up smoking in the control group is 11%.
- The percentage absolute risk reduction (ARR%) is 7%.

- The NNT is $\dfrac{1}{ARR\%} = 14$.

This means that only 14 people would need to be given nicotine replacement to cause one person to stop smoking.

QUESTIONS ON NNT

QUESTIONS

1. Explain what is meant by an NNT of 20 for the use of aspirin plus streptokinase in the treatment of acute myocardial infarction.

Your answer ....

2. The West of Scotland Coronary Prevention Study (WOSCOPS) trial was a study of coronary heart disease prevention [The WOSCOP study group West of Scotland prevention study: identification of high risk groups and comparison with other cardiovascular intervention trials. *Lancet* (1996) 348: 1341]. It assessed the rates of death for acute myocardial infarction in 6595 men aged 45–64 with raised cholesterol. The following results are taken from the published data:
The risk of cardiovascular heart disease in men aged 45–64 with plasma cholesterol levels of 6.5–8.0 mmol/l:
Placebo – 9.3%
Treatment – 6.8%
(a) Calculate the absolute risk reduction as %.
(b) Calculate the NNT.

Your answer ....

3. A review of the literature was conducted to assess the benefits of treating hypertension in the elderly [Sanderson S. Hypertension in the elderly: Pressure to treat? *Health Trends* (1996) 28: 71–74]. In the over 65s, it was found that the NNT to prevent a stroke was 22. If the same treatment was given to people under 65, would you expect the corresponding NNT to be higher or lower? State your reasoning.

Your answer ....

QUESTIONS ON NNT

Answers

Answer to question 1

This means that for every 20 patients with an acute myocardial infarction given thrombolysis and aspirin, one death would be prevented.

Answer to question 2

(a) ARR% is 9.3% – 6.8% = 2.5%

(b) The NNT is $\dfrac{1}{2.5\%} = 40$

Answer to question 3

You would expect a greater NNT in hypertensives under 65. This is because the prevalence of cerebrovascular accidents is much higher in the older age group.

SCREENING

- This chapter covers the basic principles of medical screening. The characteristics of screening tests and screening criteria are described. Questions 1−4 are numerical-type questions, whereas questions 5−8 touch on some of the ethical issues involved.

INFORMATION ON SCREENING

Screening is concerned with the secondary prevention of disease. Primary prevention will stop a particular problem or disease from occurring. Secondary prevention aims to detect a disease as early as possible or when it is asymptomatic.

> Screening investigates an apparently healthy population in order to identify asymptomatic or unidentified disease.

Screening tests are not meant to be diagnostic. Those individuals who have a positive screening result then have to undergo a further diagnostic test; for example, cervical cytology is followed by colposcopy in selected cases.

Only certain diseases are suitable for screening. A screening procedure should fulfil certain criteria. These criteria, sometimes known as 'Wilson Criteria' were drawn up by Wilson and Junger for the World Health Organisation in 1968 [Wilson J.M.G., Junger G. The principles and practice of screening for disease. *Public Health Papers*, 34. Geneva: WHO, 1968; 26–39] These criteria are shown below.

SCREENING CRITERIA

- An important **public health** problem.
- The natural history of the disease should be understood.
- Treatment at an early stage should be of more benefit than treatment started at a later stage.
- There should be a suitable test.
- The test should be **acceptable** to the population.
- There should be adequate facilities for diagnosis and treatment.
- For diseases of insidious onset, screening should be repeated at intervals determined by the natural history of the disease.
- There should be a **recognizable** early stage.
- The chance of psychological harm to those screened should be less than the chance of benefit.
- The cost of a screening programme should be balanced against the benefit it provides.

Before starting a screening programme, the characteristics of the actual screening test need to be assessed. Sensitivity, specificity and predictive values provide ways of assessing the characteristics of a screening test.

SENSITIVITY AND SPECIFICITY

The results of a screening test can be shown in a 2×2 table.

		Disease present		
		Yes	No	
Test positive	Yes	A	B	(A + B)
	No	C	D	(C + D)
		(A + C) = True positive	(B + D) = True negative	(A + B + C + D) = Total population

Sick and Fit may help you remember the definitions.

- Sensitivity is the proportion of true positives who are correctly identified by the test: $\dfrac{A}{(A+C)}$

- Specificity is the proportion of true negatives correctly identified by the test: $\dfrac{D}{(B+D)}$

As sensitivity increases, specificity decreases. A highly sensitive test could then falsely identify healthy people. Low specificity may not be acceptable if the subsequent diagnostic test is a major invasive procedure. This would mean that too many patients with a false positive result would undergo unnecessary interventions.

PREDICTIVE VALUES

The number of cases picked up through screening can be measured using the predictive value.

- The **positive predictive value** is the proportion of patients with a positive test who are correctly identified as having disease: $\dfrac{A}{(A+B)}$

- The **negative predictive value** is the proportion of patients with a negative test correctly identified as disease-free: $\dfrac{D}{(C+D)}$

These predictive values are dependent on the prevalence of a disease in a given population as well as the sensitivity and specificity. Testing for a rare disease will lead to a low positive predictive value, regardless of how high the specificity is. Another way of looking at it is if the screening population is at low risk from the disease, any positives picked up by the test are more likely to be false positives. Screening high-risk populations will increase the predictive values.

Example

In a population of 1000, the prevalence of the disease is 1%. This means that 10 people have the disease and 990 do not.

If a test has 100% sensitivity and 95% specificity, we can calculate the positive predictive value from our 2×2 table.

		Disease present		
		Yes	No	
Test positive	Yes	10	50	60
	No	0	940	940
		10 = True positive	990 = True negative	1000 = Total population

The positive predictive value is $\dfrac{10}{60} = 17\%$.

Increasing the prevalence to 2% leads to the following table:

		Disease present		
		Yes	No	
Test positive	Yes	20	49	69
	No	0	931	931
		20 = True positive	980 = True negative	1000 = Total population

The positive predictive value is now 29%.

QUESTIONS ON SCREENING

QUESTIONS

1. Define sensitivity, specificity and predictive value.

Your answer ....

2. A new test was applied to a population of 600. It correctly identified 80 of the 100 people with the disease. It picked up a further 50 people as positive who did not have the disease.

(a) What is the prevalence of the disease?
(b) What is the sensitivity of the test?
(c) What is the specificity of the test?
(d) Calculate the positive and negative predictive values.

Your answer ....

3. There are a range of tests available for screening for prostatic carcinoma:

    ● Direct rectal examination
    ● Trans-rectal ultrasound scanning
    ● Prostate-specific antigen

The sensitivity and specificity are tabled below [Davies, T. Chapter 17 in Stevens, A. (ed.) *Health Technology Evaluation Research Reviews.* Wessex Institute of Public Health Medicine.]

Type of screening test	Sensitivity	Specificity
Direct rectal examination	70%	95%
Prostate-specific antigen	80%	85%

If the prevalence of carcinoma of the prostate is 3% in the general population, calculate the predictive values for a direct rectal examination in a population of 2000. Assume that this test is used in isolation.

Your answer ....

4. Now calculate the positive predictive value for prostate-specific antigen.

Your answer ....

SCREENING PRINCIPLES

Early detection and treatment should lead to improvements in survival, not just simply 'bringing forward' of the diagnosis. Proper trials should be conducted in order to demonstrate that 'true benefits' are gained from the screening process.

5. In practice, screening for prostate cancer with prostate-specific antigen leads to two out of three men with a false positive test. Using this information and the WHO criteria, outline the main reasons against screening for carcinoma of the prostate at present.

Your answer ....

6. Screening for ovarian cancer requires that screened patients undergo diagnostic laparotomy. What are the implications of increasing the sensitivity of current screening tests?

Your answer ....

7. What outcomes would you expect to see from an effective screening programme for breast cancer?

Your answer ....

8. What are the pros and cons of genetic screening for a recessive carrier state?

Your answer ....

QUESTIONS ON SCREENING

Answers

Answer to question 1

See introductory text on pp. 106–108

Answer to question 2

		Disease present		
		Yes	No	
Test positive	Yes	80	50	130
	No	20	450	470
		100 = True positive	500 = True negative	600 = Total population

(a) $\dfrac{100}{600}$ or 1 in 6 = 17%

(b) $\dfrac{80}{100}$ true positives = 80%

(c) $\dfrac{450}{500}$ true negatives = 90%

(d) Positive predictive value is $\dfrac{80}{130}$ = 62%

Negative predictive value is $\dfrac{450}{470}$ = 95%

Answer to question 3

Positive predictive value is $\dfrac{42}{139} = 30\%$

Negative predictive value is $\dfrac{1843}{1861} = 99\%$

		Disease present (prostate cancer)		
		Yes	**No**	
Test positive (enlarged prostate)	**Yes**	42	97	139
	No	18	1843	1861
		60 = True positive	1940 = True negative	2000 = Total population

Answer to question 4

Positive predictive value is $\dfrac{48}{339} = 14\%$

		Disease present (prostate cancer)		
		Yes	**No**	
Test positive (raised PSA)	**Yes**	48	291	339
	No	12	1649	1661
		60 = True positive	1940 = True negative	2000 = Total population

Answer to question 5

- Although this is an important public health problem, the ability of current tests to detect prostate cancer without diagnosing too many false positives is poor.
- Early detection with prostate-specific antigen has not been shown to lead to an improvement in survival.

- Many men with prostate cancer are at an age when they are more likely to die of another disease.
- The available treatments (e.g. transurethral resection of the prostate, TURP) have uncertain benefits and certain effects on morbidity and mortality.
- Proper trials are needed.

Answer to question 6

Increasing the sensitivity will lead to a drop in specificity. This would result in an increase in the number of false positive patients. These patients would have to undergo diagnostic laparotomy. It would be better to maintain a high specificity to prevent this.

Answer to question 7

If we take effective to mean a beneficial outcome for the target population, we would include:

- Adequate uptake of the test.
- Good coverage of the target population.
- A reduction in the stage of cancers at diagnosis.
- A reduction in stage-specific mortality.
- An improvement in survival over 5 years.

Answer to question 8

- Genetically inherited diseases are often rare but severe.
- Genes often interact with environmental factors to cause disease, so the tests may not be a certain predictor of the future.
- There may not be an effective treatment.
- There are psychological consequences of knowing you are a carrier of a 'faulty' gene.
- Some couples have religious and ethical objections to termination of pregnancy, regardless of their genotype.
- There are issues of confidentiality if other relatives are invited to be screened.
- There are the wider implications of poor employment prospects and insurance cover to be considered.

PART III

- Quick revision section

QUICK REVISION SECTION

- On the eve of the exam, you may not have time to read through the bulk of this book. This section has been written as a quick-glance revision aid, to remind you of the bare essentials required for the critical reading section of the exam.

STUDY DESIGN

Two main types:

- Observational studies
  - (a) Cross-sectional
  - (b) Case control
  - (c) Cohort

  Strength of evidence

  ↓

- Experimental studies

  Randomised/controlled trials

  INCREASING

Cross-sectional (or prevalence studies)
- 'Snapshot' health profile
- Requires a good survey instrument
- Cannot prove cause and effect

Case-control
- Good for rare diseases
- Quick, cheap
- Gives odds ratios
- Problems of bias

Cohort
- Good for rare exposures
- Can calculate disease incidence directly
- Less bias
- Expensive
- Lengthy follow-up
- Loss of follow-up can affect validity

Randomised controlled trials
- Provide best evidence
- Random allocation to treatment or control
- Balances out confounders
- Ethics

CRITICAL APPRAISAL

Introduction	• Background
	• Aims
	• Relevance
	• Originality
Methods	• Design
	• Outcome measures
	• Subjects
Results	• Understandable
	• Response rate
	• Drop-outs
	• Statistical analysis
Discussion	• Critical evaluation of results
	• Conclusion
	• Applicability
Others	• Title, Author, Institute, Journal
	• Writing style
	• Ethics
	• References
	• Conflicts of interest

Meta-analysis appraisal	
Screening question	• Important and focused issue
	• Appropriate studies used
Methods	• Inclusion of all important studies
	• Databases searched
	• Unpublished data
	• Non-English publications
	• Personal contact with experts
	• Quality of studies assessed
	• Explicit criteria
	• Broadly similar studies combined
Results	• Bottom line result with confidence intervals, NNT
Discussion	• Applicable to general practice, costs?

GUIDELINES

Guideline development
- Assign guideline development group
- Identify key question/s
- Perform a systematic search for evidence
- Analyse evidence and compile an evidence table for each key question
- Construct recommendations based on the evidence
- Compile a draft set of guidelines and send them for external review
- Publish guidelines
- Make plans for review/update of guidelines

Critical appraisal
(1) Assemble 2–4 appraisers
(2) Appraise the following 6 domains
- Scope and purpose
- Stakeholder involvement
- Rigour of development
- Clarity of presentation
- Applicability
- Editorial independence

Positive points
Guidelines can improve the process of care and the outcome of care.

Negative points
Guidelines do not replace knowledge and skills.
They may be biased.
Different organisations use different systems.
They are only good if they are used and regularly updated.
Qualitative studies have no role in guideline development.
Issues of greatest clinical importance may be overlooked.

RISK

Risk measurements of association between exposure and outcome

Absolute risk: The background incidence of disease in the population

Relative risk: Disease incidence in the exposed population **divided by**
Disease incidence in the non-exposed population

Attributable risk: Disease incidence in the exposed population **minus**
Disease incidence in the non-exposed population

Absolute risk reduction (ARR): Proportion of treated group with desired outcome **minus**
Proportion in control group with desired outcome

NNT: The number of people who need to be treated to get desired outcome

$$\frac{1}{\text{Absolute Risk Reduction as a \%}}$$

SCREENING

Screening investigates an apparently healthy population in order to identify asymptomatic or unidentified disease

- Screening selects people for diagnostic tests
- Can be physically and psychologically harmful
- WHO criteria are a guide to the principles of screening
- Test characteristics are assessed through:

  (a) Sensitivity: The proportion of true positives identified
  (b) Specificity: The proportion of true negatives identified
  (c) Predictive values:

  - **Positive   The proportion with a positive test who are correctly diagnosed**
  - **Negative   The proportion with a negative test who are correctly diagnosed**

The success of screening programmes should be evaluated through trials

AUDIT

- Required standard: criteria for success

- Measure and record findings or performance

- Compare with standard

- Define and implement change

- Review and repeat cycle